Women Physicians

Women Physicians

Careers, status, and power

Judith Lorber

Tavistock Publications
New York and London

First published in 1984 by
Tavistock Publications
733 Third Avenue, New York, NY 10017
and
11 New Fetter Lane, London EC4P 4EE

© 1984 Judith Lorber

Typeset by Activity Limited, Salisbury, Wilts.
Printed in the United States of America

Library of Congress Cataloging in Publication Data
Lorber, Judith.
  Women physicians.

  Bibliography: p.
  1. Women physicians.   2. Women physicians——United States.
3. Women physicians——Employment——Social aspects.
4. Sexism in medicine.   I. Title.   [DNLM: 1. Physicians,
Women——United States.   2. Education, Medical——
United States.   3. Women's Rights.   W 21 L865w]
R692.L63   1984   610'.92'2   84-16213
ISBN 0-422-79040-0
ISBN 0-422-79050-8 (pbk.)

British Library Cataloguing in Publication Data
Lorber, Judith
  Women physicians: careers, status and power.
  1. Women physicians——United States
  I. Title
  331.4'8161'0973   R692

  ISBN 0-422-79040-0
  ISBN 0-422-79050-8 Pbk

Contents

For Matthew

Acknowledgements

For financial help with the research and writing, my thanks go to the Association of American University Women for the Alice Freeman Palmer Fellowship and to the Professional Staff Congress/City University of New York Faculty Research Award Program for three grants.

George Reader, MD, and Margaret W. Hilgartner, MD, facilitated the collection of data for the interview study, as did Robert Jones for the Association of American Colleges study. They have my thanks for all their help. I also owe much gratitude to the physicians who generously gave their time and thoughtfulness to the interviews.

For their perceptive reviews and critiques of parts of the manuscript, I would like to thank Mary E.W. Goss, Barbara Grenell, Charlotte Muller, and Joyce Wallace. For their careful work at various stages in the research and production of this book, I thank Martha Ecker, Nina Fortin, Nancy Naples, and Anita Redrick.

I especially thank Barbara Katz Rothman for loving emotional support, rational professional advice, a careful reading of the entire manuscript, astute editing, and most of all, for persuading me to present my convictions courageously.

It is customary at the end of the acknowledgements to thank the intimate others who, through encouragement or forbearance, made the work possible. This book is dedicated to my son because he is a very important person in my life, but it owes its existence, shape, and substance to my sisters in feminism.

New York City
February 29, 1984

Preface

Ten years ago, one of my students in a medical sociology class wrote a paper reviewing the literature on medical education in the United States. In an attempt to reverse the standard sexist language of the time, she used the pronoun "she" in place of "he" when she summarized the studies. I received a jolt on reading her paper, since my recollection was that there had been no women subjects in *Boys in White, The Student Physician,* or any other major study of physicians. My own review of these works confirmed my initial reaction – the major studies of medical education in the United States were all on men, as was the classic analysis of physicians' career development through patronage and sponsorship by Oswald Hall. The only study of medical education which included women was Emily Mumford's *Interns,* and the only extended published study of twentieth century women physicians at the time was Carole Lopate's *Women in Medicine.*

Since then, there have been numerous studies of men and women in medical training and a plethora of articles on the differences in income, productivity, and career constraints of male and female physicians. It is clear from these newer studies that while women are better represented in all specialties than they had been in the past, women medical students are still being encouraged to go into traditionally female specialties – pediatrics, family medicine, and obstetrics and gynecology. It is also clear that once in practice, women physicians, while highly productive and working continuously, are still rarely represented in the higher circles of the medical establishment – as heads of medical schools, hospitals, large research institutions, and prestigious clinical departments. Although most of the studies are of physicians in the United States, reports on women physicians in other countries show that despite differences in the proportion of female to male physicians, and in the organization of medical care, similar career patterns persist for women.

The unanswered question for me was, what aspects of the medical profession and the organization of medicine have been keeping twentieth-century women physicians from the top echelons of their profession, and will this discrimination continue? In the United States, the numbers of women in medical school increased during the 1970s to about 25 per cent, where it has leveled off. The prediction is that these greater numbers will solve the problem of women physicians' "invisibility." However, even where women physicians are already a quarter, a third, or even a majority of the medical profession, as in the Soviet Union, they are not found in similar proportions in positions of authority. They therefore have little chance to make an impact on the priorities and values of the medical care systems in which they work.

While this book is an analysis primarily of the careers of women physicians in the United States, its findings about the hidden processes of gender discrimination are probably generalizable to the experience of women physicians in other countries. Indeed, many of these processes have been found in other occupations and professions in the United States. Gender discrimination is a pervasive and tightly woven structure that is for the most part impervious to individual actions. Yet the opposite side of this coin is that social patterns are constructed out of and maintained by individual actions. The data in this book are presented in the hope that they will allow both men and women to question, and perhaps change, the taken-for-granted assumptions and decision-making patterns that structure their own and their colleagues' careers.

Chapter 1
SISTERS IN THE BROTHERHOOD:
women as professional colleagues

"The colleague group is ideally a brotherhood; to have
within it people who cannot ... be accepted as brothers
is very uncomfortable."
(E.C. Hughes)[1]

Modern women physicians present an intriguing series of puzzles. In some countries, such as the United States, they have been rare, and the stereotypical physician embodies supposed manly characteristics – rationality, objectivity, technical authoritativeness, and aggressiveness in the face of emergencies (Fidell 1980; Davidson 1978; Kosa 1970). In other societies, such as the Soviet Union, women physicians are in the majority, and the stereotypical physician embodies purported womanly characteristics – personal involvement, compassion, maternal authoritativeness, and patience in the face of long-term illness (Haug 1976).

The gender-typing of specialists also presents contradictions. In the United States, women are urged to enter either specialties with high interaction with patients, such as pediatrics or psychiatry, because such specialties are felt to be compatible with their interest in people, or they are steered into low-interaction specialties, such as pathology, anesthesiology, and public health, because the practice hours are compatible with family responsibilities (Weisman *et al.* 1980; Wunderman 1980; Davidson 1979; Grenell 1979; Ducker 1978; Quadagno 1976; Kosa and Coker 1971). Whether women are a small or large percentage of physicians, the gender concentration in the different specialties is remarkably consistent from country to country, with pediatrics the typical women's specialty and surgery the typical

1

men's (Elston 1980, 1977; Rosenthal 1979; Lapidus 1978; Leeson and Gray 1978: 33–48; Piradova 1976). In Latin America, the Middle East, and Asia, women gynecologists and obstetricians are necessary because of the modesty of female patients (Gallagher and Searle 1983; Blumberg and Dwaraki 1980; Segovia and Elinson 1978; Chaney 1973; Papanek 1971). In the United States, in the nineteenth century, similar Victorian ideas gave women physicians a competitive edge, which they completely lost in the science-minded twentieth century (Morantz 1978; Wertz and Wertz 1977; Shryock 1966). With the advent of the feminist quest for women's control over women's bodies, obstetrics and gynecology are once again thought of as a woman's specialty (Ruzek 1978).

Another area of inconsistency is the differential rewards for performance during medical training. Modern medical schools are standardized in curriculum and universalistic in their standards of accomplishment. Women enter medical schools with qualifications equal to those of men (N. P. Roos, Gaumont, and Colwill 1977; Fruen, Rothman, and Steines 1974; Nadelson and Notman 1974), and do consistently well on the tests that are the benchmarks of medical education (Holmes, Holmes, and Hassanein 1978; Johnson and Sedlacek 1975; Weinberg and Rooney 1973; Jeffreys, Gauvin, and Guleson, 1965). Yet later in their careers, women are underrepresented in the upper echelons of the medical profession. Whether women physicians are in the minority or the majority, these well-qualified professionals are rarely found running the most prestigious clinics, hospitals, or medical schools in any country.[2]

The conventional explanations for women physicians' lesser professional status have been their commitment or relegation to family responsibilities, and their lesser motivation to achieve high status. These are linked explanations, since it is inferred that women's restricted professional aspirations are the result of their choice of family over career as a lifelong commitment (Bourne and Wikler 1978). Further, it is assumed that commitment to family is a decision made early in adult life, and one which therefore circumscribes later career opportunities. However, an equally plausible explanation is that women turn to a culturally approved use of time as they are gradually shut out of career opportunities, just as men turn to community, voluntary, and sometimes even family activities when their careers are not so successful.

Whatever the timing, the data on the relationship between the professional productivity of women physicians and their marital status and number of children are not consistent. While married

2

women physicians with children do show fewer hours worked and more career interruptions than male physicians, it is not clear that their overall or lifetime productivity is less than that of men.[3] Nor is there a direct relationship between marital status or between number of children and professional productivity (P.A. Roos 1983). But most important, professional productivity is not the only, and not always the most significant, factor influencing professional status.

Women physicians' overall lack of representation in the top levels of medical institutions has also been attributed to their modest ambitions (Horner 1972). Studies which tested for success-avoidance in women found many situations in which women were ambitious – for instance, when competing with women, or for advancement in women's fields.[4] Research on women in male-dominated fields found that women could be equally competitive with men, given the right work environment (Kanter 1976, 1977a: 129–63; Epstein 1981: 175–218). It is the situation that produces ambition, not the other way around, so that women and men who are placed in challenging jobs tend to be more ambitious than those who are in dead-end work.

Explaining the lesser professional status of women by their own choices or by their own productivity assumes that career development is under the total control of the individual, and dependent only on the individual's attitudes, motivations and performance. It is an achievement model that is ideologically rooted in the presumption of equality of opportunity, fair evaluations, and reward by merit. It is an ideology increasingly coming under question. Research on male career development has underscored the importance of the structure of organizational opportunities and the help and hindrance of colleagues, patrons, mentors, and wives. So too, an adequate explanation of the underrepresentation of women physicians at the top levels of the medical profession must consider the effects on their career development of the structure of medical training and medical practice, the sorting and sifting process of sponsorship and patronage, and the help and hindrance of colleagues, mentors and husbands. These factors are better able to explain men's successes and failures than a putative merit system, and it is these factors that must also be examined for the source of women physicians' success or lack of it. Women's supposed commitment to family is part of the expectations of others, the "cultural mandate," that influences the perception of potential sponsors as to the professional worth of women (Bourne and Wikler 1978; Coser and Rokoff 1971). A woman's choice to devote her energies to her family rather than to her work may be the result, rather than the cause, of her diminished career opportunities, just as her

3

supposed lack of ambition may be the product, not the producer, of her blocked career advancement.

Interactive processes, not individual talents and choices, still keep women physicians in their supposed appropriate place. This place is the *middle* – even for those women who are qualified by virtue of training and achievement, and who have the ambition to be in positions at the very top of the profession. A woman internist in her fifties said of the women of her generation:

> They are not visible. The problem with women internists is that there are many of them who do "menial" jobs, who work in general medical clinics, and do things that are not visible intramurally or extramurally. Many of them must be excellent, and they could do fantastic jobs if they were given the opportunity on a professorship level and department chairman level. They probably don't know themselves how much of the potential they have because they weren't given the opportunity. They are hidden.

Despite their increase in number, I feel women physicians' capabilities to be heads of teaching hospitals, large medical centers, and prestigious research institutes are *still* hidden by persistent and pervasive gender discrimination.

The gender discrimination that keeps competent women physicians hidden occurs in other professions, in the sciences, and in bureaucratic organizations, and has not disappeared with the advent of the current women's movement (Epstein 1981, 1970b; Reskin 1978a; Kanter 1977a). It is rooted in the status of women in male-dominated society, and in the expectations that surround that status. Because of these expectations, women are not given the opportunities to accumulate the resources that build up careers. They are kept from the best opportunities, I feel, through a combination of rebuffs and lack of whole-hearted encouragement from those who are in a position to help their career development. This book will analyze the general social patterns that limit most women's careers, using women and men physicians as examples.

Status expectations and the Matthew effect

The theory of status expectations suggests that diffuse statuses, such as gender, significantly affect social interaction by limiting the opportunities for performance, particularly in positions of authority, of those of devalued status.[5] Those of higher status are assumed to be competent and are automatically accepted for leadership roles; those of lower status have the burden of proof – they must establish their competence and their legitimacy as potential leaders.

Status expectations are a version of the "Matthew effect": the process of accumulated advantages and visibility described for Nobel scientists by Robert Merton and Harriet Zuckerman (H. Zuckerman 1977; Merton 1968). As attributed to Christ by the Gospel according to Matthew in the King James version of the Bible, the Matthew effect reads:

> For whosoever hath, to him shall be given, and he shall have more abundance: but whosoever hath not, from him shall be taken away even that he hath. Therefore speak I to them in parables: because they seeing see not; and hearing they hear not, neither do they understand. (xxv, 29)

Christ, of course, was referring to the accumulation of faith. Merton, and others who have used the quotation similarly, was referring to the accumulation of social advantages. The second part of the quotation, on the invisibility of the process, is usually omitted, but it is an intrinsic part of the process of accumulation of advantages, in that those in positions of power, authority, privilege, and wealth, as well as those doubly deprived, usually accept the inequities as legitimate. Particularly in achievement-oriented societies, where the talented and motivated individual is supposed to have the opportunity to transcend the bonds of family, social group, and class, accumulated advantages are considered the rewards of merit and superior performance in an open competition with universalistic standards (Offe 1977; Sennett and Cobb 1973).

The Matthew effect is seen as fair.[6] There is serious question, however, as to whether competition in any field is strictly open, whether achievement alone is the main evaluative criterion, and whether the standards are objective or applied even-handedly. In short, in looking at the hierarchy of positions of power and prestige in the various work worlds of modern society, we may not be looking at meritocracies.

In most work and professional groups, both the standards and opportunities for achievement are controlled by the dominant members, who seek to preserve their ideas and values by choosing those like themselves to carry on their work. Homogeneity in a colleague group may be based on class and educational background, gender, race, religion, or ethnic group (E.C. Hughes 1971: 141–50).

5

There are communities of professionals who trained together and who choose successors from the same schools (Epstein 1981, 1970b; Freidson 1970b; Goode 1957). In teaching hospitals and research laboratories, "invisible colleges" prevail, and consensus on quality of work is heavily influenced by the evaluators' theoretical perspectives (Cole, Cole, and Simon 1981; Latour and Woolgar 1979; Mitroff 1974; S.J. Miller 1970; Crane 1972).

In medicine, which is dependent on peer regulation, the twin processes of sponsorship and boycott are at the heart of the sorting process that results in professional networks that are homogeneous on competence and ethicality (Freidson 1970b: 185–201). The acceptable novice physician becomes a protégé of a member of the élite group of established physicians, and thus gets referrals of patients, secures affiliation with the community's most prestigious hospitals, and is offered partnerships and other valuable colleague associations (O. Hall 1949, 1948, 1946). The initial probationary sponsorship makes a new physician visible to colleagues and gives him or her a chance to demonstrate competence and adequacy of performance.

If protégés were chosen by sponsors strictly on the basis of their potential, as demonstrated by their performance during training, the system *would* be based on merit. However, the choice of colleagues and successors is also usually made on the basis of other criteria, such as race and gender. In medicine in the United States, élite medical groups have tended to be made up primarily of white, Protestant men (J.E. Blackwell 1981: 73–108; Solomon 1961). When affirmative action programs urge the deliberate inclusion of race and gender as evaluative criteria for hiring and promotion, there is a feeling of uneasiness at the violation of what is supposed to be a merit system. Yet the results of previous years under this same system belie the claim that choices of protégés, colleagues, and leaders were made strictly by merit, unless the members of minority races and women were generally not as competent as white, Protestant men. Overt discrimination based on the seeming lack of competence of members of minority races and women is no longer publicly acceptable. However, gender and racial inequality still exist. Women and minority physicians are still not represented in the élite inner circles of the medical establishment in numbers proportionate to their numbers as experienced, competent, professionals. In terms of the Matthew effect, they are have-nots.

Professional gatekeepers

Gender inequality is produced and sustained by the same process that stratifies the medical profession in other ways. The heart of the process is sponsorship and patronage, and the tendency to offer opportunities for advancement to those most similar in background to the members of already established inner circles.

In medicine, evaluations are based not only on technical performance as physicians, but also on ability to get along with patients and colleagues, for these are seen as vital aspects of a doctor's work. Social characteristics, such as religion, race, ethnicity, social class background, and gender, are supposedly predictive of interpersonal behavior. The informal screening of novices uses not only medical criteria, such as accuracy of diagnoses and appropriateness of treatment, but also the purported traits of members of the various religions, races, ethnic groups, social classes, and genders. Those whom the established members of a medical community are most likely to value as future members of their inner circle are usually those who are most like them in values, demeanor, upbringing, and appearance, since these similarities are felt to be most likely to produce colleagues they can trust.

Evaluation on the basis of social characteristics, and the distributions of resources and rewards to those acceptable to the "gatekeepers," is not a malicious conspiracy, nor a pattern peculiar to medicine. It is a pervasive and persistent social phenomenon that can be found in every profession and occupation. The tendency for people to choose colleagues they can trust is rooted in the nature of work and its written and unwritten rules. Everyone at one time or another bends or breaks the rules, and everyone makes mistakes. In order to preserve a united front, colleagues look for "brothers." Everett Hughes described the process very well:

> Part of the working code of a position is discretion; it allows the colleagues to exchange confidences concerning their relations to other people. Among these confidences one finds expressions of cynicism concerning their mission, their competence, and the foibles of their superiors, themselves, their clients, their subordinates, and the public at large .... In order that men may communicate freely and confidentially, they must be able to take a good deal of each other's sentiments for granted. They must feel easy about their silences as about their utterances. These factors conspire to make colleagues, with a large body of unspoken understandings, uncomfortable in the presence of what they consider odd kinds of fellows.
>
> (E.C. Hughes 1971: 145–46)

In sum, in evaluating the job performance of novices and peers, the criteria of judgment are not only how well the person works, but whether or not the person is a trustworthy and loyal colleague. It is here that differences in race, religion, ethnic group, social class, education, and gender loom so large. In periods when group differences are taken for granted and publicly accepted, there need be no justification for rejection of a member of a "wrong" group. However, when group differences are minimized and discrimination is not socially acceptable, and may even be illegal, justification for rejection is likely to be more varied and personalized. As Goffman says of gatekeepers' decisions:

> deciders, if pressed, can employ an open-ended list of rationalizations to conceal from the subject (and even from themselves) the mix of considerations that figure in their decision and, especially, the relative weight given to these several determinants.

> (Goffman 1983: 8)

It is my contention that male gatekeepers do not yet believe that women are trustworthy colleagues, either because of their supposed characteristics or because of their competing family roles. As a result, except for the few tokens who are granted honorary manhood, most women do not become members of the powerful and prestigious inner circles that determine values, standards, and conditions of work. The current period has opened many opportunities to women, and legal and formal barriers to their advancement have fallen, but I claim that through the informal organization of work, they are still tracked mainly into lower or middle level careers.[7]

Sponsorship and the Salieri phenomenon

Women of proven competence usually do not attain a level of reward that men of similar accomplishments often receive. It is almost taken for granted that women have to be better than men to attain the same status, and what's more, there's research to prove it (Pugh and Wahrman 1983). The achievements of professional women do not build into reputations equivalent to those of similarly accomplished men, and even where their work is perceived as equally good, they are not given the promotions or prizes that men of their caliber get.[8] The failure to get their just rewards may be due to women's unfamiliarity with the game of self-presentation (Piliavin 1976), to their not maintaining helpful connections in their professional communities

(Granovetter 1973), or to their inability to negotiate themselves into positions of centrality in the organizations in which they work even when they have achieved high formal rank (Olson and J. Miller 1983, J. Miller, Lincoln, and Olson 1981).

I would argue that behind these interpersonal "failures" of women of accomplishment and aspirations is the subtle denigration of their worth by their male colleagues, by men in the larger professional networks, and even by women who want to maintain their "queen bee" status. This process is often invisible to the recipients and frequently unconscious on the part of the perpetrators, particularly when merit and performance are supposed to be the prevailing evaluative criteria. It was far more open in societies based on patronage, and so I turn to a fictional account based on such a society to illustrate what I call "the Salieri phenomenon."

In Peter Shaffer's play, *Amadeus*, Mozart's distasteful lack of social graces gives Salieri, the court composer and gatekeeper of musical patronage, the opportunity to prevent the young musician's extraordinary accomplishments from receiving recognition. Salieri recommends Mozart to the dispenser of patronage, the Emperor Joseph, but makes sure that the rewards he gets are minimal. In the process, Salieri pretends to be a benefactor of Mozart, and the blocking of Mozart's career advancement is hidden from him. Here is the Salieri phenomenon in action:

[EMPEROR] JOSEPH: We must find him a post.
SALIERI: ...There's nothing available, Majesty.
JOSEPH: There's Chamber Composer, now that Gluck is dead.
SALIERI: (Shocked). Mozart to follow Gluck?
JOSEPH: I won't have him say that I drove him away. You know what a tongue he has.
SALIERI: Then grant him Gluck's post, Majesty, but not his salary. That would be wrong.
JOSEPH: Gluck got two thousand florins a year. What should Mozart get?
SALIERI: Two hundred. Light payment, yes, but for light duties.
JOSEPH: Perfectly fair. I'm obliged to you, Court Composer.

And here is the response from the unwitting victim, who is persuaded he has been helped by a powerful patron:

MOZART: It's a damned insult. Not enough to keep a mouse in cheese for a week!...
SALIERI: I'm sorry it's made you angry. I'd not have suggested it if I'd known you'd be distressed.

9

MOZART: You suggested it?
SALIERI: I regret I was not able to do more.
MOZART: Oh...forgive me! You're a good man! I see that now!
You're a truly kind man–and I'm a monstrous fool!
(Shaffer 1980: 71–2)

Salieri was generous with his tutelage and patronage to those composers whose musical talents were the equivalent of his, such as Gluck, or who were clearly his junior, such as Beethoven. His meanness to Mozart was to a potential rival who was not only of superior talent, but whose new ideas challenged Salieri's musical hegemony. The importance of the Salieri phenomenon is that it is used not just against all newcomers with unacceptable traits or social backgrounds, but against those who might establish new standards. These upstarts' ideas would break the chain that links patron to protégé and that upholds the values and beliefs of the current establishment. Patronage is not withheld from those who are willing to assimilate, but it is not likely to be granted to those who would make the patron obsolete.

The Salieri phenomenon sets in motion a circular process. Those of devalued status get less opportunity to show what they can do, and when they do perform well, their work is undervalued. As a result, they get a smaller share of rewards and resources. Fewer rewards and resources (the negative aspect of the Matthew effect) means diminished power, authority, and prestige. The resultant diminished *achieved* social standing reinforces the initial devalued *ascribed* social status and perpetuates – and justifies – the established stratification system. In modern times, the Salieri phenomenon is used in recommendations for positions, promotions, and officerships in professional associations, in reviews and in citations of published work and work-in-progress, and in professional shoptalk that evaluates the competence of colleagues.

To the extent that reputation in any field reflects ascribed social statuses and personal and political maneuverings on the part of the person and his or her status evaluators, there can be no objective worth based on universalistic standards. Performance and behavior are judged by those who dominate the inner circles, and their standards are likely to mirror their own values and those of the social group to which they belong. Their power and control of resources are brought to bear on those who are ambitious to achieve high status, but only those who will not challenge the gatekeepers' values are given serious opportunities to compete. Mozart's unacceptable social behavior laid him open to Salieri's denigration of his work and ruin of his professional reputation until long after his death, when his music could be judged separately from him as a person and its perceived quality assessed by a different musical community with new standards. Unfortunately, while alive, he suffered from poverty and lack of visibility.

Women's double binds

Women suffer from a series of ironic double binds that virtually guarantee that they will not be fully accepted members of their predominantly male colleague communities. If they are married, they are considered committed to their family, rather than to their career (Lorber 1979; Osaka 1978; Bourne and Wikler 1978; Coser and Rokoff 1971). If they are unmarried, they are considered unreliable or dangerous protégées and colleagues, because the assumption is that a sexual relationship is their prime priority (Kaufman 1978; Reskin 1978a; Epstein 1970a: 965–82, 1970b). If their lesser resources as bosses make them resort to a conciliatory style, they are considered to be too soft to be effective leaders (Martin and Osmond 1982). If they choose a leadership style that is socially distant and task-oriented, they are felt to be too inflexible to be successful supervisors (South *et al*. 1982; Kanter 1976).

Nurturant, emotional, and supportive women are tracked into lower prestige work and not considered leadership material, but aggressive women are also heavily penalized because of the implied threat to men's dominant position. If self-advancement is seen by men as aggressive, those women will be devalued as *women* and hence become socially unacceptable to the very men who can help them (Brown and Klein 1982). But if women are soft-spoken and reticent, they are likely to be overlooked. Whatever interactive stances women assume are likely to defeat their bids to become members of male-dominated inner circles, let alone leaders of these groups (Epstein 1981, 1974a: 265–302; Wolf and Fligstein 1979a; Reskin 1978a; Wolman and Frank 1975).

Status expectations theory predicts the near impossibility that, as individuals, those of devalued status will break through the stereotyped values that keep them down. If the devalued overachieve to compensate for the discounting of their accomplishments, they may be regarded as selfish and unconcerned with the needs of the group. If they make a bid for leadership, their behavior is seen as

11

inappropriate and is ignored or penalized. If they try to appeal to a superior for help and documentation as to their trustworthiness and worth to the group, they must demonstrate their social acceptability. But their social acceptability usually depends on their displaying characteristics that reinforce the initial devalued status. Even if the devalued status is neutralized in a particular colleague community, the person involved is not likely to attain credence easily in a new colleague group, particularly if it is a larger or higher circle of power. Until the evaluation of the whole group changes, any one individual who tries to break out suffers from what Everett Hughes called the dilemmas and contradictions of status (E.C. Hughes 1971: 141–50).

Career development of female and male physicians

To what extent are women physicians affected by the Matthew effect and the Salieri phenomenon? How do their careers differ from those of their male peers? I analyzed the careers of a matched sample of men and women who had entered medical school in 1956, and who had been followed through 1976 (see Appendix I). I found that despite good performance and high evaluations in medical school, and internship at prestigious teaching hospitals, women physicians did not sustain their early accomplishments. By mid-career, their professional attainment lagged behind men with similar initial performance, but the survey data could not tell me why.

In order to uncover the processes that shape physicians' careers, I conducted in-depth interviews with sixty-four female and male physicians who were affiliated with the Department of Medicine of a prestigious metropolitan medical center (see Appendix II). The interviews lasted one to two hours, and covered the physicians' training, past and current work situations, choices made, interpersonal influences, relationships with colleagues and patients, effects of family life, main professional accomplishments, plans for the future, and regrets for past decisions. The interview data documented what produced the differences in men's and women's careers – limited sponsorship for women after the early career stages, and taken-for-granted inequality in the family division of labor even for women physicians married to physicians. Both the process and results of career development for women and men physicians have been found for women and men in other occupations and professions (Rossiter 1982; Epstein 1981, 1970b; Poll 1978; Reskin 1978b; Kanter 1977a; Bernard 1964). Women physicians should not be seen as unique, but rather as a prototype of highly qualified women who are trying to attain equal status in a male-dominated work world.

This book compares the career development of men and women physicians who practiced in the United States between 1940 and 1979. Their careers cover three periods: the first, one of open discrimination against women in admissions to medical school, in restriction of internships and residencies, and in prejudice from patients; the second, a period of transition when overt discrimination became illegal and women were admitted to medical schools in growing numbers; and the third, a period where about one-quarter of the students in medical school were women, voluntary and enforced affirmative action opened more staff, practice and research opportunities to women, and the feminist movement encouraged women to seek out women physicians.

Attitudes toward women were not the only changes in the medical profession during this time. The 1940s and 1950s were a heyday of autonomy, prestige, and expansion of the medical profession. In the 1960s, heavy capital investment in high technology equipment led to the growth of large, centralized medical empires, and the expansion of services encouraged increasing government penetration through tax-based funding and payment plans. The 1970s brought shrinking financial support from the government, the emergence of cost-cutting regulation, and the beginning of bureaucratic incorporation of hospitals and physician groups under private capitalization (Starr 1982). Women entered medicine in the United States in greater numbers as the profession's prerogatives and prestige diminished (Carter and Carter 1981).

From the point of view of everyday routines and relationships, however, remarkably little has changed. With patients and with ancillary health care providers, physicians were and still are the dominant profession (Freidson 1970a). Among colleagues, a patronage or sponsorship system has operated continuously to stratify what is supposed to be a merit system. Oswald Hall found in the 1940s that through personalized evaluations and advancement, physicians in a community organize themselves into a series of homogenous concentric circles – an inner élite, a "friendly," less powerful, outer circle loosely tied to the most powerful and prestigious physicians, and isolated loners (O. Hall 1949, 1948, 1946). Hall found that those novice physicians whose performance, demeanor and social characteristics were acceptable to the established physicians were sponsored for advancement. Through a graduated series of resources and rewards, such as referrals, hospital privileges, partnerships, staff appointments, and organizational memberships, the favored new physicians are set on the path to becoming members of the powerful and prestigious inner circles of community physicians. While the locus of professional power has shifted in the last decade from the community physician to the hospital-based physician, no matter what the type of career, the pattern of advancement is still along the lines of sponsorship and patronage (A.E. Miller 1977).

The rest of the book will show the effects of this system on the women and men I interviewed. But first, I want to make clear the place of professional patronage and sponsorship in the overall organization of medical services, and how it impinges on women and men at different times in the profession's history.

Notes

1 E.C. Hughes 1971:148.
2 For the United States, see Jolly 1981; Farrell *et al.* 1979; Wallis, Gilder, and Thaler 1981; Wilson 1981; Witte, Arem, and Holguin 1976. For England and Wales, see Leeson and Gray 1978; Elston 1977. For Australia, see Fett 1976. For Sweden, see Frey 1980. For the Soviet Union, see Lapidus 1978; and Dodge 1971. For cross-national comparisons, see Rosenthal 1979.
3 See Ward 1982; Ducker 1980; Heins and Braslow 1981; Mandelbaum 1981 and 1978; Nadelson, Notman, and Lowenstein 1979; Yohalem 1979; Quadagno 1978; P.B. Williams 1978; Elston 1977; Heins *et al.* 1977; L.K. Cartwright 1977; Heins *et al.* 1976; Cohen and Korper 1976; Fett 1976; Jussim and Muller 1975; Bewley and Bewley 1975; J.G. Jones 1971.
4 See Kaufman and Richardson 1982: 30–59; Garland and Smith 1981; Intons-Peterson and Johnson 1980; Tresemer 1977, 1976; Makosky 1976; Levine and Crumrine 1975.
5 See Pugh and Wahrman 1983; Humphreys and Berger 1981; Webster and Driskell 1978; Berger *et al.* 1977; Berger, Cohen and Zelditch 1972; Epstein 1970a.
6 See J.R. Cole 1979. For a challenge to this view, see Martin 1982 and Tuchman 1980.
7 As Freidson (1970b: 201) said, "while the sorting and sifting of cooperative colleague relations...is deliberate and conscious enough, its organized outcome is largely neither acknowledged nor recognized *as organization* by its participants" (emphasis in original).
8 Documentation for this statement can be found in Ahern and Scott (1981) and in J.R. Cole (1979). Cole, however, insists that the scientific establishment is fair, and that status is based on productivity. His main

criterion of scientific worth is citations of published work, which he uses as an objective measure of visibility. As Martin (1982) says in her critique of *Fair Science*, visibility, perceived quality of work and citations to that work are probably not separate variables, but "it is entirely possible that all three are indicators of the single concept 'social status' of the scientist" (p. 492). For an extended account of the unfairness of the scientific establishment to women, see Rossiter (1982).

Chapter 2
A RESERVE ARMY:
women physicians and the
organization of medicine

"Was there no way to nip the bud of ambition without
cutting off the supply of necessary workers?"
(*Kessler-Harris*)[1]

Women physicians, like other women workers in both capitalist and
communist countries, are likely to be found in less prestigious,
lower-paid work (Coser 1981; Treiman and P.A. Roos 1983). Women
have access to work in occupations that are not of high priority in
commanding economic resources and where the workers are relatively
powerless politically; women are restricted in their opportunities for
work in occupations or professions that command prestige and high
income, and where the workers have control over the conditions and
terms of their work. Medicine's openness to women physicians has
varied with the strength of the profession and with the demand for
lower cost doctors. Women's supposed prime commitment to family
responsibilities justifies restricting their access to work of higher
reward, but they are encouraged to enter the labor force where there is
a shortage of male workers. Women's actual commitments, interests,
and motivations are of less importance in their patterns of work than
their society's need for certain kinds of workers. In this sense,
women, including women physicians, are a "reserve army."[2]
Before the nineteenth century, there was no medical profession in
the sense of a group of workers with similar training, way of working,
and reliable clientele, but there were periods where some physicians,
with the support of powerful members of society, were able to
monopolize the more lucrative clientele. Once physicians began to
consolidate their control of the delivery of medical services, the means
of restriction became more extensive (Larson 1977). Women

16

physicians' opportunities shrank with the success of the physicians' project to become a full-fledged profession, but have expanded again as physicians are coming under various forms of regulation. The question for the future is whether women physicians' status and power will be equivalent to that of male physicians, or whether, in an increasingly constricted profession, women physicians will find themselves in the lower ranks.

Pre-nineteenth century:
"Worthless and presumptious women who usurped the profession"[3]

Throughout the greatest part of human history, most people had bones set, boils lanced, teeth pulled, fevers brought down, babies delivered, and limbs amputated by lay healers, who were either self-taught, or had learned their skills and medicinal lore from other lay healers. These healers were themselves aristocrats, peasants, and even slaves, and of course, women as well as men (Morantz 1982b; Wertz and Wertz 1977; Morais 1976; Ehrenreich and English 1973; Bullough and Bullough 1972; M.J. Hughes 1943). Periodically, the observations and skills of a few of these healers were written down for posterity, and their names and knowledge are therefore available to us. These, too, include women, such as Trotula, the eleventh century author of a major treatise on the diseases of women (Ehrenreich and English 1973; M.J. Hughes 1943; Hurd-Mead 1931).

As Western Europe became more urbanized in the eleventh and twelfth centuries, the first universities appeared and medicine was taught formally. Although literate women had as much access as literate men did to the Greek and Latin texts on which university medical training was based, such as those by Galen and Hippocrates, the universities themselves were generally closed to women. For male university-trained doctors, the cost of their education could be offset only by the fees paid by urban, upper-class patients. In an attempt to monopolize this clientele, and to maintain a superior status, these physicians, with church support, charged that non-university trained physicians, especially women, were practicing illegally, and brought several to trial (Ehrenreich and English 1973: 15–16). In England, physicians petitioned Parliament to impose fines and imprisonment on the "worthless and presumptuous women who usurped the profession" (Ehrenreich and English 1973: 17). Urban, educated male doctors restricted the paid medical practices of urban, educated women, particularly among those of their own class, but they could not stop these same women from healing their families, retainers, and servants.

Lay healers who could heal where university trained doctors could not were frequently accused of witchcraft, the argument being that if those who had their learning under church auspices were unsuccessful, unauthorized cures must come from collusion with the devil.[4] However, neither witch hunts nor licensing of only those with university training eliminated lay healers.[5] Since only upper-class women and men could afford the fees of the formally trained physicians, the mass of the population was treated by female and male local lay healers, who were frequently paid in goods or services, and who did not have the status, such as it was, of formally trained physicians. The knowledge and skills of the lay healers remained unrecorded and localized, and they, in turn, had limited access to the theories, observations, and instruments of the formally trained physicians. As the body of scientific medical knowledge and practice grew, lay healers became increasingly isolated and vulnerable to legal restrictions.

Nineteenth century medicine:
"I had no medical companionship"[6]

In the nineteenth century, medical practice in Europe remained stratified on class lines (Elston 1980, 1977; Larson 1977; 80–103). Only those physicians who had the patronage of the aristocracy had a modicum of professional status. In the United States, geographical mobility and the absence of a hereditary aristocracy created a more open structure, in which women, blacks, and those without much wealth or social position could gain a minimal formal medical education. During this period, sectarian physicians competed with traditional or "regular" doctors, and on all sides practices were clustered around persuasive purveyors of medical beliefs. The regulars and the sects, with different notions about the causes of illness and appropriate cures, ran their own schools and dispensaries, and had their faithful following (Rothstein 1972).

In this atmosphere, any claim that attracted clients and maligned the competition was fair. Women physicians were able to get medical training at the sectarian schools of lesser prestige, but they were

18

excluded from the "regular" medical schools, whose more authoritative degrees could have countered the stigma of their gender (Morantz 1982b; Walsh 1977: 1–34). The few women who did manage to gain admission to these schools, and therefore had an education equal to that of their male competitors, were then ostracized by the medical societies that controlled consultant referrals, and were not allowed to practice in the dispensaries and clinics run by the regular physicians. Given the openness of the organization of practice and the common clusters of like-minded physicians and patients, women were able to compensate for their excommunication by forming female-dominated medical circles and by turning Victorian ideas about "true womanhood" to their own ends (Morantz 1978; Walsh 1977: 76–105; Drachman 1976).

Elizabeth Blackwell, the first American woman physician to attend an East Coast regular medical college, complained that once trained, she still was not welcome as a member of the medical community in New York City. She said, "I had no medical companionship, the profession stood aloof, and society was distrustful of the innovation.... I was advised to form my own dispensary" (E. Blackwell 1977: 190). And so she did, later inviting her sister, Emily, and Dr Marie Zakrzewska to join her on the staff of the New York Infirmary for Women and Children. Opened in 1857, it was the first woman-staffed hospital in the United States. It was followed by the New England Hospital for Women and Children, founded by Dr Zakrzewska in Boston in 1862. These dispensaries were financed by wealthy women who served as trustees, and who formed the better paying clientele of the women physicians who ran them. In comparison to the trustee-dominated all-male Boston Lying-In Hospital, the women trustees of the New England Hospital for Women gave the women physicians a freer hand with administration and finances, and so they were able to provide a better quality of care. Even though their ideas on therapeutics were similar to those of their male colleagues, they kept careful records for all patients, not just those of the middle class, varied length of stay by social need, and used hospital design that minimized the spread of puerperal fever (Morantz and Zschoche 1980; Walsh 1977: 76–105).

For American women physicians as well as men, success in the nineteenth century lay in attracting a circle of wealthy and socially prominent patrons and in setting up their own networks of schools, hospitals, and dispensaries (Starr 1982: 89–90). Although American women physicians were accepted as members of medical associations in the latter part of the century, they formed their own medical societies

19

as well, consolidating their associations with each other and with the educational societies of their female patrons (Marrett 1980, 1979). These female-dominated institutions, Walsh has pointed out, formed "an island of feminist strength and sisterhood in a society only familiar with brotherhood" (Walsh 1977: 103). Women physicians supported and symbolized the movement for equal rights for women, and the feminists, in turn, helped establish women physicians' rights and opportunities. As Walsh said:

> The women's rights movement called for female physicians as a matter of principle, stimulated fund-raising and scholarships, and promoted feminist institutions.... Equally important, feminism furnished women with the moral and psychological support that enabled them to function in a culture generally hostile to feminine achievement.
>
> (Walsh 1977: xvi)

However, female separatism, the ideology of feminine modesty, and women physicians' claims to special affinity for the care of women and children were two-edged weapons (Morantz 1982b, 1978; Shryock 1966). They gave women doctors a competitive edge during a time of cut-throat entrepreneurship, but when women wanted to be included in the upgrading of medical education and to share in the increasing power and prestige of the physicians, the ideology of sex differences was used against them (Walsh 1977: 178–206; Bullough and Voght 1973; Smith-Rosenberg and Rosenberg 1973). The financial contributions of women philanthropists were substantial enough to force the new Johns Hopkins Medical School to agree to admit women "on the same terms precisely" (McPherson 1981), but women's social power was not great enough to ensure the admission of more than a small number of women. When all but one of the women's medical schools were closed in the widespread reform of medical education at the beginning of the twentieth century, only a few women physicians found places in the new, upgraded medical schools, and even fewer were admitted to hospitals for further training. Mary Putnam Jacobi's optimistic prediction on hearing that Johns Hopkins would be coeducational turned out to be partly right and ironically wrong. She said:

> The admission of women to share in these higher opportunities is a fact of immense significance, though only a few should profit by the advantage, the standing of all will be benefited by this

authoritative recognition of a capacity in women for studies, on this higher plane, on equal terms and in company with men.
(Quoted in B.J. Harris 1978: 108)

Women physicians as a whole did benefit from the greater standing of the emerging dominant medical profession, but they were neither treated equally with men nor did they share men's company as colleagues.

Twentieth century medicine: "On the inside sitting alone"[7]

The upgrading of medical education in the twentieth century produced practitioners who were more scientifically trained and clinically experienced than those of the nineteenth century, but it also restricted legal medical practice only to those holders of the MD degree and those health workers under MD authority. For the first time in Western history, lay workers were rejected by the populace, who were more and more persuaded of the efficacy of modern medicine, as practiced by MDs, through a growing series of drugs, vaccines, anesthetics, and surgical procedures. Knowledge of modern medicine was widely disseminated through public health campaigns, the routine examination of school children, and free well-baby care for poor families (Starr 1982: 180–97). With the encouragement of the American Medical Association, muckraking propaganda against non-licensed healers and patent medicines further damned sectarianism, self-medication, lay midwifery, and folk healing (Starr 1982: 123–44; Kobrin 1966). Legal medical practice was brought under the control of one group of professionals, who now monopolized access to training, clientele, hospitals, and clinical research. To trace the position of women physicians in the twentieth century, one must look at differences in the organization of medical work, which I will do for the United States, England, and the Soviet Union.

UNITED STATES

In the United States, the twentieth century saw a shift from client-controlled practices dependent on the whims and beliefs of patients to colleague-controlled practices dependent on the good opinion and reciprocal favors of other physicians (Freidson 1960). Not only did established physicians determine who got into medical school, what they studied there, and whether they were competent to practice, but the same inner circles of physicians controlled the selection for specialty training programs, making it possible to locate novice physicians on the basis of gender, religion, race, and ethnic group into "appropriate" types of practices.

The prestigious, research-oriented, and better paying specialties were reserved for white, Protestant, upper middle-class men. Obstetrics and gynecology, a lucrative specialty until the late 1960s, was heavily male once midwifery was driven underground. General surgery and specialty surgery, which command high fees and have developed a charismatic aura, are almost exclusively male. Pediatrics, pathology, public health, anesthesiology, radiology, and dermatology accepted women, Jews, Catholics, blacks, and, after World War II, foreign medical graduates into their training programs. Industrial and occupational medicine was of such low status that, in 1918, when Harvard wanted to hire someone to teach it, the only qualified candidate was a woman physician, Alice Hamilton. Harvard hired her, but she was not allowed to march in the commencement academic processions, was not allowed into the faculty club, and was never promoted, in fifteen years, above assistant professor (Walsh 1977: 211–12).

Control by powerful colleague groups continued after training and, unlike medical school admissions, was unmitigated by state intervention. As gatekeepers of hospital privileges and referrals of patients, the established physicians in a community determined future physicians' career advancement. Discrimination by race and ethnic group was so widespread that Catholic, Jewish, and black doctors encouraged their respective philanthropic societies to endow hospitals, so that they would have places to train, staff appointments, and beds for their patients. Their alternatives were the municipal hospitals, with access controlled by urban political bosses (Starr 1982: 173–74).

The power of the local colleague group was enhanced by the rules of liability in malpractice suits, which were set in the late nineteenth century as the standard of care in the local community of physicians. The locality rule limited expert testimony for and against a physician to immediate colleagues. Local medical societies promised to defend their members and were able to get low malpractice insurance rates for them, while doctors who did not belong had a hard time getting any insurance at all (Starr 1982: 111–12). Thus, as Starr says, "the local medical fraternity became the arbiter of a doctor's position and fortune, and he (sic) could no longer choose to ignore it" (Starr 1982: 111).

As early as 1904, Dr Bertha Van Hoosen felt that the women who attended the American Medical Association's annual meeting were isolated and ineffectual. She said, "A generation earlier, women doctors were on the outside standing together. Now they were on the inside sitting alone. Their influence was nil" (quoted in Walsh 1977: 213). However, with concerted pressure, their influence could still be brought to bear on at least one issue – maternal and child health.

After World War I and the victory of female suffrage, women reformers helped pass the Sheppard-Towner Act, which, in 1921, set up state and federally funded prenatal and child health centers throughout the country (S.M. Rothman 1978: 136–53). They were staffed and directed by female physicians and public health nurses, who offered preventive care, hygiene education, and low cost medical services in the best tradition of the ninetenth-century women's dispensaries. But by 1929, the American Medical Association coopted preventive care for the private physician and led the fight to deny further funding for the Sheppard-Towner clinics. The 1930 White House Conference on the Health and Protection of Children was dominated by male physicians (Costin 1983). After 1930, faced with the Depression and World War II, and handicapped by low numbers, geographical isolation, the power of the American Medical Association, and the waning of active feminism, women physicians faded into virtual invisibility (Lorber 1975a).

American women physicians from the 1930s to the 1950s may have found it easier to assimilate than to build their own networks and institutions, as Jewish, Catholic, and black male physicians did, because they tended to be recruited from the upper middle classes and to attend the prestigious women's colleges that were the counterparts of the Ivy League schools of their white, Protestant, male colleagues (Lopate 1968: 31–33; P.A. Williams 1971). The women's upbringing, education, and family ties may have made them acceptable as "friendly" colleagues, as long as they did not assertively counter the open discriminatory practices that permeated medical education and practice during this period.

Also important in dampening their ambitions was the "cultural mandate" – the supposed need of the family for the mother's commitment to its concerns, a commitment that was held to outweigh any professional commitment (Bourne and Wikler 1978). As Kessler-Harris says of the women workers of the post-World War I period:

To induce women to take jobs while simultaneously restraining their ambition to rise in them requires a series of socially accepted constraints on work roles. Unspoken social prescription – a tacit understanding about the primacy of home roles – remained the most forceful influence. This is most apparent in professional jobs where the potential for ambition was greatest.

(Kessler-Harris 1982:231)

Rossiter (1982) details this process for women scientists.

In the 1960s, under the impact of the civil rights movement and the new feminist consciousness, overt discrimination in education, hiring, and promotion was outlawed, and careers for women met with more public approval. The 1960s also saw a jump in third-party reimbursements, and a consequent rise in demand for physicians' services. The women physicians of this transition period tended to act on their own to further their careers, seeking out medical institutions that were most open (or least hostile) for training and staff positions. They made the most of limited sponsorship (Lorber 1981a).

The youngest cohort of women physicians in the United States are still at the beginning of their careers. They have two advantages. As junior physicians, they are least threatening as colleagues, and most likely to receive the help of established male senior physicians. They also have more senior women to turn to for mentorships and sponsorship, active women's professional organizations, and a new feminist movement for support, attitudinal change, and clientele. But if the senior women do not garner resources to distribute to the junior women doctors under their wing, and the men who still dominate the upper echelons of national and community medical institutions do not become more amenable to grooming women as their successors, these younger women, too, may find that their accomplishments do not bring them the ranks and statuses equal to those of their male peers.

Medical work in America is coming more and more under government and corporate regulation. Large-scale tax-supported medical institutions, such as teaching and research centers, overshadow the prestige and political power of the local community practitioner (A.E. Miller 1977). With primary care and specialty practice paid for by third-party insurance payments, governments and profit-oriented corporations are imposing cost-cutting regulations (Starr 1982: 420–49). Before speculating on how these developments may affect women physicians' careers in the United Sates, I will discuss how the organization of medicine affected women physicians' careers in England under the National Health Service and in the

24

Soviet Union, where medicine is completely under state control. While neither medical system is likely to be replicated in the United States in the near future, some lessons might be learned from women physicians' experiences under systems of prepaid office practices and salaried clinic and hospital positions.

ENGLAND

Women physicians in England, like those in the United States, were recruited from the upper middle classes, encountered similar quotas in medical schools, had relatively powerless national and provincial women's medical associations, were underrepresented in policy-making bodies, and expressed dissatisfaction with the progress of their careers (Elston 1980, 1977; Leeson and Gray 1978). Although the power of the profession was located in national and regional councils, rather than in the local community colleague group, women physicians' careers in England were similar to those of their American counterparts. They were relegated to low-paying, low-status specialties, and were offered more opportunities for work in primary care than in hospital consultantships.

The plans for the National Health Service in 1944 recommended coeducation for all English medical schools and the admission of a "reasonable" proportion of women students. Although the ceiling was set at 20 per cent, the actual quota was 15 per cent, the pre-World War II national average. The women who went to medical school, as in the United States, tended to be better qualified than the men because of the restrictions on their numbers.

The quotas were abolished in the late 1960s, when there was an expansion of hospitals and an increased demand for, as Elston puts it, "pairs of hands," especially in the less popular specialties and in the peripheral hospitals. As in the United States, the lower-grade positions and the less prestigious specialties tended to be staffed by women and foreign-trained physicians. Women are half of the physicians in community medicine, family planning clinics, and child health. These fields are underfinanced and of lower prestige than the surgical specialties and hospital consultantships, where women hold a tenth of the posts (Leeson and Gray 1978: 37–8).

The central planning and careful structuring of the medical labor supply under the National Health Service relegated women physicians to the less advantageous sector of what is essentially a dual labor market (Elston 1977). The higher paying sectors, with open career ladders and stable demands for workers, have been reserved for Anglo-Saxon males, while women and foreign-trained MDs are

25

generally found in the secondary sector, which is characterized by lower pay, blocked upward mobility, and fluctuating demand for workers. While women's family commitments and interests are used as the rationale for this internal segregation, a better explanation is the demand for low-cost medical workers. Given their underrepresentation in the policy-making councils of the National Health Service and the British Medical Association, women physicians became an exploitable reserve pool of inexpensive medical labor.

SOVIET UNION

The status of women physicians in the Soviet Union seems to be the complete antithesis of that of American women doctors. Because men were in short supply after World War I and the revolution, women are the majority of the profession. Their numbers in medical schools went down, rather than up, in the 1960s in order to achieve parity for men students (Lapidus 1978: 188). They are salaried employees in community and work enterprise polyclinics, where their duties are preventive as well as curative. Haug notes that "they get to know the workers well, check on their health, follow up those with chronic conditions, lecture on health matters, and monitor compliance with safety and health rules" (Haug 1976: 98). In the neighborhood polyclinics, women physicians are very much part of the social scene, and their relationship with patients tends to be maternal and solicitous rather than objective and scientific (Haug 1976: 98). Soviet physicians' relations with patients are not entirely benign, as their mandate is to keep the labor force at work.

The domination of the medical profession by women indicates that it is not one of high economic priority, since the work women do in the Soviet Union is routinely paid less than the work men usually do (Swafford 1978). Not only are physicians not a powerful occupational group, but within medicine, women physicians do not dominate the positions of power. Even though three-quarters of Soviet physicians are women, they are only half the directors, deputy directors and chief physicians in clinics and hospitals (Dodge 1971: 218).

Women in general are underrepresented on the national levels of Communist Party membership and activity, the chief avenue to power in the Soviet Union. Again, their own motivations and family responsibilities (despite institutionalized child care services) are given as the reason for their low political participation. But, as Lapidus points out, "... within the Party itself there is considerable hesitation in promoting women to positions of real authority" (Lapidus 1978: 227).

The work and professional status of women physicians in the Soviet Union resemble that of the women doctors in England who staff the community health, family planning, and child health clinics. Similar medical workers in the United States are public health nurses and family care nurse practitioners, and school and employee health service physicians, all of whom tend to be female. In all three countries, low-paid, low-prestige women health workers carry the bulk of primary, preventative, and routine care – the everyday, unglamorous work of medicine.

The overall situation of women physicians in all three countries is more alike than different despite the dissimilarities in the organization of medical work, which is entrepreneurial and collegial in the United States, government controlled and locally coordinated in England, and state planned in the Soviet Union. And, in all three countries, women physicians are absent, as professionals and as ordinary citizens, from the corridors of power.

Twenty-first century medicine: "The peak of the pyramid?"[8]

In the United States, physicians, including women physicians, are at the top of the pyramid of health-care workers. The crucial issue is whether the status and power of women physicians will rise commensurately with their increase in numbers, or whether, like women physicians in England and the Soviet Union, they will increasingly find themselves doing mainly primary and preventive care. These vital areas of medical work bring women doctors in competition with other women health workers, particularly nurse practitioners, who claim expertise in the same areas of health care (Lurie 1981). If nurse practitioners also offer diagnoses and treatment of routine illnesses and preventive care, and offer it at lower cost, women physicians will be hard pressed to claim superior status or payment. And yet, it is as primary care practitioners that the new women physicians are being "welcomed" into the profession (Geyman 1980; Relman 1980; Wallace 1980). A typical statement is as follows:

> The women's groups in the United States now trying to take steps to improve women's health care are the consumer, nurse midwives, and nurse practitioners. One would expect women physicians to be in the vanguard of this movement, but this is not the case. Similarly, one would hope that the care of women of the

27

childbearing age and the care of infants and children would be delivered together. Thus, women physicians have a unique opportunity and role to play in improving the system by delivery of health care in the United States. This should be one of the top priorities for women physicians for today and tomorrow.

(Wallace 1980: 211)

Would such a mandate give women physicians a powerful position in medicine? Only if family health care had top priority in funding, and women doctors were given the authority to organize and direct these services. In the United States, under entrepreneurial practice, when services become lucrative, they are taken over by male physicians (Pawluch 1983). In England, under the National Health Service, this sector of medical care is underfunded (Elston 1977). In the Soviet Union, where extensive primary and preventive care is mandated by the state, women physicians have authority over patients, but not over state medical policy (Lapidus 1978; Haug 1976).

In the United States, as medical practice becomes more bureaucratized under government and corporate control, women physicians will probably be overrepresented in the rank-and-file of provider institutions.[9] Rather than forming the vanguard of a consumer-oriented, open-access medical system, women physicians are likely to find themselves in competition for autonomy, status, and even jobs with nurse practitioners, nurse midwives, and physicians' assistants. They will all be doing virtually the same work, and professional status will lay in political power games (Lorber and Satow 1977). Such infighting makes the colleague group in the workplace crucial, and it is precisely here that women lose out (Olson and Miller 1983; Wolf and Fligstein 1979a, 1979b). With increasing numbers of doctors and growing competition from non MD licensed health workers, male physicians are not likely to forego the chance to point to women's family commitments or unsuitability for leadership in an effort to retain a competitive edge and administrative control of health care delivery institutions and academic medicine. Under pressure from outside, the colleague group can be expected to close ranks against competitors, and for male physicians, these competitors may very well be women physicians.

In the near future, women physicians in the United States are likely to split into two groups: those who align with other physicians in the fight to maintain professional dominance, and those who align with other women health-care workers and consumers in the fight for a health care system with a flatter hierarchy and a holistic and self-help perspective (Howell 1977; Kleiber and Light 1978; Ruzek 1978; Shapiro and A.B. Jones 1979). As with so much else about women physicians, their opportunities and dilemmas mirror the structured choices and political strategies of other women workers in their respective societies. Their elite professional position in the United States makes them an excellent test case for the chances of women in an individualistic, capitalist society, for if women in a prestigious, highly paid profession can't make it to the top, which women can? The women physicians in England and the Soviet Union are also important object lessons for women physicians, for they demonstrate that national planning and funding and state control, in the absence of a built-in structure for gender equality, end up being just as exploitative as entrepreneurial collegiality.

Notes

1 Kessler-Harris 1982: 230.
2 See Rosenthal and Eaton 1982; Elston 1977. As a reserve army, women physicians compete with foreign-trained doctors (see Goldblatt and Goldblatt 1976). A combination of both low-prestige statuses – female and foreign – limits the career opportunities of Soviet women physicians who emigrate to Israel. Primary care in community clinics is the typical work of Israeli women physicians, who comprise 25 per cent of all physicians and 42 per cent of community clinic practitioners. Soviet immigrant physicians of both sexes tend to end up in such practices, but more men than women are eventually licensed for hospital practice. The women Soviet physicians, who are 64 per cent of the immigrant group, are more satisfied with their positions in Israel than the men, despite a heavy work load in the community clinics, perhaps because their status at least replicates where they stood in the Soviet Union (Shuval 1983).
3 Ehrenreich and English 1973: 17.
4 Ehrenreich and English 1973: 12–17. On the "white witch" as healer, see Szasz 1970.
5 A literary account of the dangers of a women's lay healing can be found in Shakespeare's *All's Well That Ends Well*. Helena, "a poor unlearned virgin, is careful to attribute her possession of the cure for the king's longstanding malady to her late father and to legitimate its efficacy by *his* learning and skill, "the greatest of his profession." Even so, the king is afraid of being ridiculed if he submits to her ministrations. He says:
   "We thank you, maiden,
   But may not be so credulous of cure,
   When our most learned doctors leave us, and
   The congregated college have concluded

29

That labouring art can never ransom nature
From her inaidable estate: I say we must not
So stain our judgment, or corrupt our hope,
To prostitute our past-cure malady
To empirics, or to dissever so
Our great self and our credit, to esteem
A senseless help, when help past sense we deem.

(Act 2, Sc. 2, 1. 115–25)

He does not allow her to try her remedy until she entreats him, "Of heaven, not me, make an experiment," and wagers her reputation as a woman, and her life, on the outcome. Her payment for success is, not unexpectedly, a high-born husband. He is loath to marry "a poor physician's daughter," but all ends well.

6 E. Blackwell 1977. Originally published 1895.
7 Walsh 1977: 213.
8 Jones and Shapiro 1979.
9 For analyses of the current structure of the health care delivery system in the United States, and predictions of the future see Freidson 1983; Starr 1982: 235–49; Mechanic 1976.

Chapter 3
MEDICAL EDUCATION:
sorting and tracking

"They have to accept you whether they like it or not"
(Woman physician)

During medical training, a group of young people whose under-graduate education and entering achievement levels are virtually identical, since they are the "cream of the crop," are sorted and tracked into differentiated colleague communities. The highly qualified, scientifically oriented, and idealistically motivated women and men who enter medical school become clinical researchers or patient focused practitioners, generalists concerned with the whole body or mind, or specialists focusing in depth on particular aspects of illness or medical care. These career outcomes are not the result of individual choice alone, but represent the sum of their choices within a limited range of opportunities (Davidson 1979).

The gatekeepers to these opportunities are the medical school faculty and the teaching practitioners.[1] During the clinical years of medical training, novice physicians are looked over by senior members of the medical community for potential partners, research collaborators, and hospital staff members. The medical students and house staff are judged not only on their professional competence, but also on their interpersonal skills. The evaluation and subsequent encouragement and discouragement by senior physicians determine to a great extent the specialties physicians in training choose, the type of practices they gravitate toward, and the career opportunities they encounter.

The tracking of students into research-oriented or patient-focused careers begins very early and is determined to a great extent by the

31

type of medical school attended, the location of postgraduate education, and faculty sponsorship (Marshall, Fulton and Wessen 1978; H.S. Zuckerman 1978; S.J. Miller 1970). Good students from academically oriented medical schools have better opportunities for further training than do good students from clinically oriented schools (Zuckerman 1978). Since type of internships and location of postgraduate training are crucial career determinants, students' choices are narrowed from the very day they enter medical school.

This is not to say that achievement counts for naught. Students' capacity for performance, as perceived by the faculty, sorts them into those who are sponsored or given particular encouragement, and those who are more or less left to fend for themselves (Marshall, Fulton, and Wesson 1978). Some of those who are ignored may later perform well enough to come to the attention of the faculty gatekeepers, but the burden of proof is on them. The sponsored students, in contrast, have a favored status from the beginning.

When it comes to the choice of specialty, both students and faculty have preconceived notions of the fit of personalities and the demands of the specialty (Ducker 1978; Fishman and Zimet 1972; Zimet and Held 1975; Gray, Newman and Rheinhardt 1966). Surgeons are supposed to be aggressive and unemotional, and pediatricians emotionally sensitive. Women physicians, especially, are supposed to have characteristics that make certain specialties, such as pediatrics and psychiatry, particularly appropriate for them. Even though the actual personalities of men and women medical students and the real practice demands of the various specialties may not fit these stereotyped notions, they are powerful influences in shaping students' choices and in determining faculty encouragement and discouragement of those choices.

The fields most frequently recommended for women are pediatrics, psychiatry, and anesthesiology. The claimed advantages of these fields for women are short training period, noncompetitive, women's sensitivity to the problems involved, ability to relate well to the clientele, and acceptance in the area. However, no one specialty offers all of these advantages, and a careful examination reveals internal contradictions in the reasons why specialties are recommended to women. For example, psychiatry has a long, not short, training period; exquisite sensitivity to the emotions of children might make treating them difficult; anesthesiology has low patient contact, and so on.

For the women themselves, perhaps the most crucial rationale is that women are already accepted in the specialty. Women students tend to choose fields where women physicians already practice, so that they will feel comfortable and welcome (Quadagno 1976).[2] Arguing that women's specialty choices are a result of positive reinforcement and conflict avoidance, Quadagno points out that this process continues to reinforce the stereotyping of certain specialties as inaccessible to women, and concludes that rather than opening up all of medicine, "the influx of women into medicine may result in increasing the sex differentiation with certain specialties becoming 'female' and others 'male' occupations (Quadagno 1976: 449).

Pediatrics and psychiatry have had a long-standing overrepresentation of women physicians, and United States data show that the attraction of these two specialties for women has not waned (Cuca 1979). The specialties that have been added to the list of favorites for women students are obstetrics–gynecology and family practice (Geyman 1980). It is questionable whether these choices reflect the students' actual preferences or their preferences after they are faced with encouragement and discouragement from the faculty. Internal medicine is the best-liked specialty for both men and women students, but many women none the less plan to go into pediatrics, and men into surgical specialties (Cuca 1979).

The men are apt to follow their preferences in their career choices; the women are not. One study showed that only a slightly greater percentage of women preferred pediatrics, compared to men, but over twice as many females as males chose this specialty (Mattesón and Smith 1977). Approximately the same percentage of men who preferred family practice chose it, but women chose this specialty almost twice as frequently as they expressed a preference for it. Two-thirds of the men who preferred surgery chose it, but only one-third of the women.

While the ostensible reason for the encouragement of women to go into pediatrics, psychiatry, and family practice, and men into surgery, is that these specialties are compatible with feminine and masculine personality characteristics (M.B. Harris and Conley-Muth 1981; Beil, Sisk, and W.E. Miller 1980), there is little evidence that women medical students are particularly nurturant and male medical students particularly aggressive. A study in which 95 female and 166 male students evaluated their own personalities found that "females rated themselves significantly higher than...males did on self-confidence, autonomy, and aggression, while males rated themselves higher than did females on nurturance, affiliation, and deference" (McGrath and Zimet 1977b: 297). Nevertheless, this same group succumbed to gender stereotyping of specialties – 69 per cent of the women intended

33

to specialize in family practice or pediatrics, but only 43 per cent of the men planned such "affiliative" careers. The result of the tracking system in medical school is that women are urged to go into specialties that tend to pay less and which are rated lower in prestige by the students themselves (Langwell 1982; McGrath and Zimet 1977b).

Helps and hindrances:
"He just sort of took me under his wing"

There are three patterns of interpersonal involvement that lead to the career option selected by the end of medical training: deliberate grooming by a faculty sponsor, role models, and being offered a congenial training opportunity. Men are likely to have a sponsor during training and to fall into serendipitous training opportunities. Women tend to pattern themselves after role models, who give only indirect guidance, rather than active help.

A senior physician who picks you out and grooms you in his or her own specialty is a powerful influence, as the following account by a woman in her forties attests:

> All along, this gentlemen was a very good friend of mine – an older man, a European. He was really my mentor, I would say. He was really the person who got me into dermatology and wanted me to be there, and he just sort of took me under his wing. I'm sure he was a very important factor – the reason I'm not doing something else. I took an elective in dermatology, and then he was very encouraging, and he wanted me to come back for another month of electives. He became a personal friend. The residency opened up. There was a space, and he urged me, "Well, come and try it for a year." So I did and it was all right.

A male physician in his thirties described in similar terms his intense wooing by two senior physicians in a small hospital where he was a resident. He said:

> Dr – made a conscious effort to interest me in gastroenterology, and he had the support of the chief of medicine. I found the two of them both excellent teachers and clinicians. They made it seem very exciting and interesting, and to some extent, they also wooed me just a little bit. Dr – took me to a meeting in Boston in the fall of that year. They took me to the national GI meeting in

Philadelphia in May and I loved it. The meetings were excellent, very stimulating. I had a good time, and that's when I decided to go into gastroenterology. I also had them behind me pushing me and guiding me into my choice of fellowships. I was starting late to look for fellowships, and it would have been difficult, but I had the two of them assisting and making entrés.

Working with a senior physician gave another male oncologist in his thirties experience that he was able to use many times in his developing career. He said:

During medical school, I was working with an enzymologist on a laboratory project. It helped me make my decision to go into medical oncology. I strangely enough used that project ever since, on and off. It helped me in reading scientific literature and understanding what research was all about. It showed me an awful lot about the difficulties, the rewards, and other things about doing research. I published a paper from it, and presented a paper about it, which was the first presentation I'd ever made. It was probably an advantage when I applied for a fellowship. The chief of medical oncology had done similar work. I think the fact that we spoke the same language didn't hurt at all.

In recognition of the worth of such experiences, a woman physician in her thirties, who did not have such help, uses only women undergraduates in her laboratory, and told her undergraduate college that she has positions available for women who are interested in science and are thinking of going to medical school.

While nowhere near as intense as direct help from sponsors, admiration (or dislike) for teachers, chiefs of service, and heads of laboratories have molded the career choices and professional styles of generations of students. One woman in her sixties said:

Probably what influences you is, obviously, whether the school is strong in that department, and also I think there are personal relationships with your professors – the ones that inspire you and the ones that leave you cold. There were two or three that absolutely made me loathe the subject I was taking.

One man in his thirties said of his role model, the chief of cardiology:

He was the hotshot. He was my role model at the time – my impressionable years. He was capable and sharp and clinically very, very smart. You had to be really on your toes to go one up on him. And when you did that you felt very happy – as he smiled cagily. He was a good model for training, and you felt you were cranked out of his mold when he put his name on your degree. I like to quote him on rounds.

Another way of making choices is coming on opportunities for training more or less accidentally. Some of these opportunities may be the result of suggestions by mentors, others are serendipitous. An example of a move that helped shape a new career direction occurred in the history of a young male researcher in his thirties. In order to stay out of the army, he got a recommendation for a research position at the US Public Health Service. Being in a research-oriented setting led to a career in academic medicine rather than his previously contemplated one in private practice. He said:

> The research I did in Washington was interesting, and so were the activities associated with academic medicine. Teaching and research became a lot more attractive than I had thought of before. I had never had any experience of it. It was sort of a forced experience and I enjoyed it. I had decided to go straight into private practice, but I went into academic medicine and spent a lot more time in research than I had originally planned when I was in medical school. Others went there wanting to do academic medicine, and then they didn't enjoy it.

Several male physicians found a place in a research laboratory through "following their noses" into interesting leads, which meant informal participation on projects others were working on, and then being asked to continue as a formal member of the group. A physician in his forties described what he had done as a resident:

> As soon as I arrived, in addition to taking care of patients, I started looking around to see who was doing things that I found interesting and worth doing. The chemotherapy group fell very nicely into that description. I started participating in their activities as a resident whenever I had time to do so, and I took elective time with them when it was available. They liked me and I liked them.

A young woman researcher arranged a training experience for herself which combined several subspecialties. She said:

> I worked out the program myself, and then a number of other people thought it was such a good idea that most of our fellows that came after have done similar things. It never got organized

into a real program, but since I had established that precedent, other people were able to do it.

In such instances, young physicians need initiative and assertiveness, and they have to be personable enough to be encouraged to continue their participation. Other situations demand flexibility in order to take advantage of an unexpected opportunity. A clinical researcher in her forties shifted her subspecialty because of the availability of a fellowship in a different, but related, field from the one she had been working in. She said:

> I had intended to do a fellowship in infectious diseases. My husband and I came here because he wanted to work in one of the units, and the infectious disease program was filled up. We had fellowships abroad in between and mine was in microbiology. The work I was doing could go either way. It could be applied to hematology. It could be applied to infectious diseases. It just so happened there was an opening here in hematology and not one in infectious diseases. I had to take the program that was open, which I think turned out to be the better program. I think it led me into a much more rewarding research field.

The choices made by the end of the training, whether for private practice or academic medicine, for a generalist practice or a narrowly focused specialty, are, in many cases, not the final step in professional options. Many physicians shift career locations, widen or deepen their medical focus, and work alternatively or successively in research and practice. These career shifts, both during and after training, are the outcome not only of their own proclivities and efforts, but equally the result of the perceptions and behavior of those they come in contact with.

On the surface, the women interviewed had similar experiences to the men during training. They had active sponsors, modeled themselves on admired older physicians, sought training opportunities, and took advantage of unexpected offers. While the men had an edge in the active encouragement of gatekeepers, the women did not seem to be seriously hindered in their early career development. But this overt equal treatment was undermined by covert instances of discrimination and devaluation.

The persistence of discriminatory policies: "The facts of life"

There is a belief among women and men physicians and the lay public that discriminatory policies in medical training are a thing of the past.

It is true that no medical schools in the United States refuse to admit women any more, and some even have entering classes that are half women. It is also true that no US medical school excludes any women from any part of their training, as did the urology departments of Johns Hopkins and Columbia in the 1940s.[3] However, as late as the 1960s, there were covert discriminatory policies against women for internships, despite a nationwide matching program of students' and hospitals' choices, as well as denials of financial support and scholarship recommendations. The details of the experience of an extremely well-qualified woman now in her forties is illustrative of the persistence of such covert policies, despite an overt system ostensibly based on merit.

This clinical researcher had been one of the top ten winners of the Westinghouse Science Talent Search in high school. She attended a prestigious medical school, where she won an award for outstanding medical research and presented her findings at a national meeting as a senior. She said:

> My first choice for internship would have been my school, but for ten years they had taken no women interns. An unspoken, unwritten policy of not taking women. I did a substantial amount of research when I was a student, and my research mentor very much supported an application for internship there. He also, though, quietly fed back to me the facts of life as they became apparent. He was unhappy that I didn't put my school down as my first choice [in the matching program], but it became clear to me that the consensus of opinion was still not to take women, and if I should be selected because of his pressure, there would still be enough unhappiness about it that I really didn't want to be the first one. I put another school down as my first choice, which then had a policy of taking one woman a year, maximally, in their medicine program, and I was chosen for it.

A woman now in her thirties was denied the nomination of her medical school for a prestigious fellowship because they had never heard of a woman getting it. That year three women did get it, and for the first time in many years, her school had no winners. Another woman in her thirties, who was one of the top students in her class, was not taken to the American Medical Association meetings, as was the practice for outstanding seniors in her school, because, she was told, there was no one she could share a room with. A woman reported being denied a salary as a third-year resident in dermatology in favor of a married man as late as the 1970s. He turned out to be divorced, and he switched to a different specialty after a year, wasting one of the few paid residencies. She felt that the moonlighting she had to do to support herself was an even better learning experience than the residency program. But in actuality, she, like the women who didn't learn to catheterize males in the 1940s, who had to settle for second-choice internships in the 1960s, who lost support for research projects and who were not introduced at professional meetings in the early 1970s, was denied a significant part of her medical training. While such overt discriminatory practices may be hard to find today, restriction of women's opportunities in medicine through the devaluation of their competence and commitment are still rampant (Bourne and Wikler 1978; Gross and Cravitz 1975; Shapley 1974).

Devaluation of women:
"Part of it isn't said with a smile"

Just as overt non-discriminatory policies are undercut by covert discriminatory practices, socially unacceptable public sexist remarks are replaced with snide comments or insinuations that are harder to confront, because, as one respondent in her thirties noted, they are said with a smile. As she put it:

> You do get a lot of so-called teasing – so-called the "what do you expect, you're only a woman" kind of stuff that people say with a smile on their face. Sometimes I think that underneath part of it isn't said with a smile. It's hard to know.

Another woman in her thirties had similar doubts about the real feelings underlying the external acceptance of women in medicine:

> There may be some background feeling about women in medicine, and that will take some time to get over. I think that as more women come in that will decrease. If you do your job well and you're confident in yourself, you can handle it fairly easily. I think if you perform adequately, then they have to accept you whether they like it nor not. Whether they like it, I don't know. Sometimes I'm not always sure about that.

What these women do not hear is what the men say to each other. One man, a cardiologist, also in his thirties, was candid enough to say:

In the coat room, there's always occasional discussion. A tearful intern – "Isn't that a pity she broke up with her boyfriend," – or this or that concerning the emotional fallibility of women. The frailty of women theme always comes out.

The belief that as the numbers of women increase, they will be more accepted by men has not been borne out by recent experiences or research. One study set out to test Kanter's theory that as women go from being tokens to being a substantial minority of a group, they will be better integrated (Kanter 1977b). The study found instead that as the proportions of women increase they have less contact with their male colleagues and get less social support from them, and also less encouragement from male supervisors (South *et al.* 1982b).

Good performance and tactful assertiveness are usually recommended as ways in which women can overcome their negative evaluation by men. However, the need to "prove yourself a little more," as a woman in her fifties put it, can be a never-ending process (Pugh and Wahrman 1983). A physician now in her sixties recounted how she got a residency at a prestigious hospital despite the fact that her interviewer had said they did not need any women, and she had to perform at an extremely high level from there on. As she said:

> The woman who preceded me had an absolutely fantastic record. She was finishing her residency, so they were still open to having women, but she was the only one they had ever had, and they expected me to be like her. All the other residents and interns were men, and a couple of them resented me because I was their boss. I remember one guy who was really very resentful of me, and would try to challenge me at every turn. Fortunately, one time I did pull a real, real smart answer for him, and from then on he never challenged me again. So I was lucky on that one.

The smart answers and superb performances can also backfire. One respondent in her thirties said that a friend of hers who was a researcher at a prestigious laboratory felt it was harder to prove yourself as a woman:

> On rounds, you have to be very careful what you say. You can't be too bright or it upsets them. She will say things and the next day, they'll be said back to her as if they came from them. There's a lot of men there with very big egos, and she ends up having to tiptoe around the egos.

40

There is a double bind of expectations, especially for young women. As physicians, it is felt they should exhibit assertive, "masculine" qualities, but as women they are then criticized for being abrasive and unfeminine (Brown and Klein 1982). These patterns are long-standing. A national sample of medical students in the class of 1960 were asked to predict which of their classmates they thought would be outstanding members of the profession (AAMC Longitudinal Survey of the Class of 1960; see Appendix I). When the composite rating scores were run against the scores on a personality test, it was found that women who rated high on achievement motivation, autonomy, dominance, and aggression were consistently less likely than the men with those personality characteristics to be considered the outstanding physicians of the future. Only women physicians with high achievement motivation alone were considered marked for success. None the less, it is the combination of these characteristics, as we have seen, that gives the training physician the best possible learning experience.

A study of residents in obstetrics–gynecology found that to get cases, do surgery, and work with the attending physicians who were good teachers and role models and who would let them operate, novice physicians needed a high level of confidence and assertiveness (Scully 1980: 198–232). Relationships with the chief resident, with senior residents, and with the attending staff were crucial to making the postgraduate years as rewarding as possible. The more naïve residents, who thought the schedules "came automatically out of heaven," were less satisfied with their rotations. There were few women in this study, but one wonders whether the women who *did* assert themselves with their superiors and peers were devalued for the very pushiness that was so valuable to the men.

Those who do not stand up for themselves often end up being pushed aside. In my study, a woman physician in her forties described the horrors her internship year presented because of her inability to handle the aggressive manipulativeness of her mostly male peers:

> I had led such a sheltered life. I had grown up in a family that took care of us. Then I went to an all-girls school; then I went to a medical school where women were treated so nicely. I don't mean we were put on a pedestal, but we weren't imposed on, weren't put upon. I went into an internship program where I was just ground down. I didn't know what hit me. It was just like being in a revolving door. I was absolutely bowled over. I had never been treated like that in my life, the way those boys treated

me. I was really overwhelmed. They were aggressive, and they just dumped the work on you, and they dumped this, and they dumped that. They took every holiday off. I worked Christmas, I worked Easter, I worked the whole goddam time. I could not wait to get out of the hospital. It was the most horrendous year of my life. I was never raised in that kind of aggressive situation, and I just didn't know what to do with it.

Times do change – a woman in her thirties described the women in her medical school as "high-powered or very ego-driven," and other women found good male friends in medical school and during their internships.[4]

In recent years, many medical schools have formed support groups and systematic networks of female faculty and students. They provide role models, mentoring, and help in facing up to overt and covert sexism.[5] Conferences and workshops which involve women students at all levels of training, as well as women faculty and practitioners, afford women at every career stage the opportunity to share experiences and coping skills.

Performance in medical training: What's the payoff?

Whatever the obstacles, women perform as well as men during their medical education (Holmes, Holmes and Hassanein 1978). I scored the doctors I interviewed on the prestige of their internship and residency hospital, whether or not they had a fellowship, and whether or not they had an award during training or had been a chief resident.[6] Given a maximum score of 6, the mean for the men was 4.54 and for the women, 4.06. For training which ranged over a forty-year period, these women and men were not far apart in their achievements. But did these achievements pay off in later professional status? Because these men and women were interviewed at different stages of their careers, it was impossible to determine whether their performance in medical training had paid off equally well in later professional attainment. For this purpose, I used the data from the national sample of physicians who graduated from medical school in 1960, and who were followed through 1976, when they were all in their forties (AAMC Survey; see Appendix I).

The women and men physicians in the national sample were matched evenly on their intellectual capacity and type of medical school. Sixteen years after graduation, the men's professional

Table 1 *Professional attainment of matched sample of physician respondents to AAMC longitudinal survey of class of 1960*

professional attainment[1]	male no.	%	female no.	%	total no.	%
low	44	15.1	33	34.0	77	19.8
moderate	194	66.7	54	55.7	248	63.9
high	53	18.2	10	10.3	63	16.2

Notes: [1]significance = .001.
  Chi Sq. = 17.27   DF = 2
  T = .1379   V = 164 (Cramer's V)

attainment was significantly higher than the women's (see *Table 1*).[7] The men's careers had progressed in a sustained way, while the women's careers had a stop and go pattern.

The men and women did equally well in medical school. Neither their scores on the National Board of Medical Examiners (NBME) test nor their ratings by faculty in their junior year were significantly different. The women were more likely than the men to have interned at relatively prestigious teaching hospitals, perhaps because more of these hospitals were beginning to open up their programs to women by 1960 (see *Table 2*).[8]

In addition to educational performance and clinical training location, achievement motivation, peer support, and family responsibilities are also supposed to affect professional attainment. On these factors, the men and women in the matched sample differed. On the personality test given to them as entering students in 1956, the men scored significantly higher than the women on achievement motivation.[9] When the medical students were asked in 1958 to predict which members of their class were likely to become outstanding members of their profession, more men than women were given high ratings. By 1976, more of the men were married and they had more children. Of the women, 28 per cent were childless. However, the women had more responsibility for household management (see *Table 2*).

All of the variables, including family responsibilities, had a positive impact on professional attainment for men. The statistically significant factors were achievement motivation, NBME score, and prestige of internship hospital (see *Table 3*). Each factor in turn had an impact on the next, in chronological order (see *Figure 1*). The male physicians who had high achievement motivation tended to have high NBME

Table 2 *Scores on independent variables for matched sample of respondents to AAMC longitudinal survey of class of 1960*

variable[1]	males		females		total	
	no.	%	no.	%	no.	%
EPPS[2]						
low score	115	39.9	50	51.5	165	42.9
high score	173	60.1	47	48.5	220	57.1
NBME examination						
low score	117	49.6	40	52.6	157	50.3
high score	119	50.4	36	47.4	155	49.7
junior-year accomplishment						
bottom third of cohort	79	28.5	25	29.4	104	28.7
middle third of cohort	104	37.5	32	37.6	136	37.6
top third of cohort	94	33.9	28	32.9	122	33.7
peer evaluations[3]						
low	143	52.4	61	67.0	204	56.0
high	130	47.6	30	32.9	160	44.0
prestige of hospital[4]						
low	111	43.4	23	27.7	134	39.5
high	145	56.6	60	72.3	205	60.5
degree of family responsibility						
low	19	6.5	25	25.8	44	11.3
medium	96	33.0	23	23.7	119	30.7
high	176	60.5	49	50.5	225	58.0

Notes: [1]significance test = Eta coefficient.
[2]significance = .02.
[3]significance = .007.
[4]significance = .01.

scores. Their peers predicted that those with high test scores and high junior-year standings would be outstanding members of their profession. Those with high NBME scores and high peer ratings tended to intern at high-prestige hospitals. High achievement motivation, good medical school performance and prestigious training location were likely to lead to a high level of professional

Table 3 *Effect of predictors on professional attainment of respondents to AAMC longitudinal survey of class of 1960*

predictors	female physicians' professional attainment		male physicians' professional attainment	
	b	beta	b	beta
EPPS score	.12	.05	.32*	.13*
NBME examination mean score	.13*	.23*	.98*	.16*
junior-year accomplishment report rating	−.22	−.07	.30	.10
peer evaluations	.21	.04	.13	.04
prestige of internship hospital	1.12*	.19*	.78*	.15*
degree of family responsibility	−.61*	−.25*	.22	.06

Note: *significant at .05 level
significant test = F test

attainment. Those men who did well in medical school tended to have fewer family responsibilities, which seems to suggest that early on, they chose a career over a family orientation. Whatever their choice, family responsibilities did not have a direct effect on men's professional attainment.

For the women, some factors were positive and some negative. Both good junior-year accomplishment ratings and a high level of family responsibilities had a negative effect on women physicians' professional attainment, but only the latter was statistically significant. The positive determiners of later professional attainment for women were NBME scores and prestige of internship hospital (see *Table 3*). Quality of postgraduate education had an even greater effect on women's professional attainment than on men's. Since a good postgraduate program offers superior opportunities for research, further training, and referrals, it can offset the stigma of women physicians' gender.

Women's career development was not consistent and progressive, the way the men's was (see *Figure 2*). For the women, high NBME scores and a prestigious training location usually led to high professional attainment, but not to recognition by faculty or fellow students along the way. They must have had faculty support to get

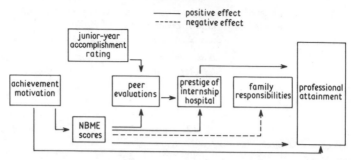

Figure 1   *Path model of statistically significant variables in male physicians' career development*

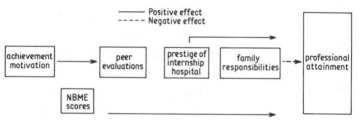

Figure 2   *Path model of statistically significant variables in female physicians' career development*

into good internship programs, but the statistical analysis does not show when this occured. Peers predicted success for women with high achievement motivation, but in actuality, this factor was not important in their eventual professional attainment. Unlike the men, the women with high family responsibilities tended to have a lower professional attainment level.

Family commitments and lack of ambition are usually targeted as the main barriers to women's professional success. The chronological career path of the women in this national sample shows that they did not get the same payoff as men from achievement motivation. They do get an important advantage from high test scores and good training location, but neither peer nor faculty recognition of their accomplishments. Given this cross-cutting of factors in their careers, women physicians may have increased their family responsibilities because of the limits on their professional attainment, rather than limiting their professional commitments because of increased family responsibilities, as is usually thought.

In sum, career development for male physicians follows a progressive and direct line, with many factors contributing to professional attainment. For women physicians, fewer factors have an effect on professional attainment, and these do not build on each other. The variables used in the AAMC study – achievement motivation, medical school performance, faculty and peer recognition in medical school, internship location, and family responsibilities – are usually cited as determinants of success, but they explained only a very small percentage of the gender differences in professional attainment. (The path models explained 13 per cent of the variance in professional attainment for men and 14 per cent for women.) Left out of the quantitative analysis are the personal helps and hindrances that shape physicians' careers before they complete their training and that are even more important as their careers develop.

Notes

1 There have been excellent studies of the socialization of male medical students into the professional community, and their relationships with faculty and senior physicians have been well documented (see Scully 1980; Coombs 1978; Bucher and Stelling 1977; Bloom 1973; S.J. Miller 1970; Mumford 1970; Becker *et al.* 1961; Merton, Reader, and Kendall 1957).

2 Epstein (1981: 101–11) found a similar process of specialty choice in law.

3 As documented by two of the interviewees, women were excluded from the lectures and clinical training in urology because they concerned male genitalia.

4 Grenell (1979) suggests that a substantial group of women medical students are ambitious and career oriented, and a substantial percentage of their male peers are family oriented.

5 See Kutner and Brogan 1981; Rinke 1981; Fesith 1977; Roeske and Lake 1977; and Hilberman *et al.* 1975. Similar women's groups can be found in law schools, according to Epstein 1981: 71–5.

6 High-prestige hospitals were teaching hospitals; medium-prestige hospitals were municipal, affiliated veterans', community, military; low-prestige hospitals were proprietary.

7 Level of professional attainment was measured by summing the following factors: board certification, publication of articles in professional journals within the last five years, presentation of papers before professional groups, administration, conducting research studies, development of medical or surgical procedures within the last five years, offices held in professional organizations, service on professional committees, referrals of patients from outside and within the physicians' own specialty, medical

school rank, and administrative position. The scores, which ranged from 0 to 12, were trichotomized as low (0–3), moderate (4–8), and high (9–12).

8 Permission to use *Tables 2* and *3* and *Figures 1* and *2* was granted by the Association of American Medical Colleges, publishers of the *Journal of Medical Education*. For an extended discussion of the analysis of the AAMC data, see Lorber and Ecker 1983.

9 The Edwards Personal Preference Schedule (EPPS) measure of achievement motivation is summarized by the following description of this factor:

> To do one's best, to be successful, to accomplish tasks requiring skill and effort, to be a recognized authority, to accomplish something of great significance, to do a difficult job well, to solve problems and puzzles, to be able to do things better than others, to write a great novel or play. (Edwards 1953)

Chapter 4
OFFICE PRACTICE:
referrals and reciprocity

"I want to make sure that the next generation gets a fair shake"
(Woman physician)

Where patients have a choice of physicians, in order to build a practice, a physician needs referrals. Referrals can come from patients who make recommendations to others on the basis of their satisfaction with their own experience with a physician. However, a novice physician without many patients cannot depend on such word-of-mouth advertising. Another way of building a practice is to work part time, doing routine physicals, and hope that some of those who need further treatment will become private patients. Usually, though, the part-time job is only an economic back-up until the office practice becomes self-supporting. A more reliable way to build a clientele is through referrals from an associate in the same office or hospital. Another good source of referrals is through former classmates in other specialties who are practicing in the same geographical area. And finally, a physician who is retiring and sells a practice usually refers the whole patient list to the doctor who takes over.

Both the patient and the colleague referral system are dependent on first-hand knowledge of the physician. When patients are shared by two physicians in different specialties, such as a gynecologist and an internist, the patient additionally becomes a source of information through expression of satisfaction or dissatisfaction with the referral, and also as evidence of each physicians' judgement and competence. Because the physician's own judgement is called into question if the patient is poorly treated, and no physician wants to inherit a botched case, referrals are not likely to continue unless both physicians' standards of competence, ethicality, and pleasantness are met. These referrals back and forth create two interrelated networks – the lay referral system among patients and the colleague referral system among physicans (Freidson 1960). Dependent as they are on personalized knowledge, subjective impressions, and particularized standards of both curing and caring, both referral networks tend to be homogeneous. Patients refer friends, relatives, and co-workers to physicians they are satisfied with, and physicians with like expectations refer among themselves. Those whose views differ usually sort out into other referral networks.

Colleague networks, referrals, and informal consulting occur not only within a community but also within medical organizations, such as hospitals and large group practices (Luke and Thomson 1980; Freidson 1975; Hummell, Kaupen-Hall, and Kaupen 1970). Whether the nexus is the referrals of patients, "curb-side" consultations, and hospital or group-practice gossip, a constant sorting, sifting, and social exchange takes place. This exchange rewards those approved by colleagues with more referrals and consultations, affiliations, and promotions, and excludes or isolates those who are not approved (Shortell 1973).

The informal organization of practicing physicians in the United States has been described as a series of concentric circles, consisting of the "inner fraternity" who control the best clienteles and the best hospital positions in a community; "friendly" physicians who are on good terms with those in the inner circle, but not an intimate part of it; and "individualistic" doctors who are highly competitive because they must hustle for patients (O. Hall 1949, 1948, 1946). Colleague networks tend to split along religious-ethnic lines, and a large city will typically have Protestant, Jewish and Catholic circles (Solomon 1961). Patients tend to come from the same religious-ethnic background as their physicians, and the voluntary hospitals where these patients are sent are supported by Protestant, Jewish, and Catholic charities respectively.

Black physicians who have been trained in predominantly black medical institutions, and who have been denied visiting privileges in all but the black teaching hospitals and in municipal, charity, or Veteran's Administration hospitals, where many patients are black, have been forced into *de facto* homogeneous colleague and patient relationships. More recently, however, blacks have sought out blacks as associates as a matter of policy (J.E. Blackwell 1981: 73–108). A similar situation of forced colleagueship has been true for foreign medical school graduates (J.G. Fox and Richards 1977; Stevens, Goodman, and Mick 1974). Women, however, have rarely banded with women colleagues, since there have usually been few women physicians in a community, and, after the nineteenth century, few women staffed hospitals. As a result, women physicians in office practice must integrate themselves into predeominantly male networks.

In my interviews with the physicians with office-based careers, I paid particular attention to what kind of help female and male physicians got in setting up an office, how they got referrals, how they related to patients, and how well they were integrated into colleague networks.

Setting up a practice:
"I know a lot of people"

The work of a young physician trying to set up a practice seems to resemble a patchwork quilt more than anything else. While the main goal is to run an office of one's own that is self-supporting and profitable on patients' fees alone, most young physicians work at a variety of jobs. They work part-time in pre-paid group practices and nursing homes; they cover for established physicians on nights and weekends; they do physicals in companies, schools, and government offices; they run emergency rooms and specialty clinics for a salary; they lend their names as medical directors or consultants to pharmaceutical companies, medical advertising agencies, and newsletters and magazines with physician audiences. The men I interviewed with office-based careers had soon phased out these early back-up jobs, and were, after several years, able to live on the income from private practice. The women with office-based careers, however, often continued to juggle practices and a mosaic of part-time salaried jobs. In the future, corporate for-profit group practices will add to the variety of possible positions, but will not reduce the reliance on colleagues for referrals to these positions (A.E. Miller 1977).

All of the positions, as well as direct referrals of patients, came to the physicians interviewed through personal contacts. A male physician in his thirties, with a practice that had just opened, was renting his office from another doctor, covering for other physicians, running a hospital emergency room, and teaching, all the while also trying to get patients. His contacts, he said, came from the medical center in which he had done training. As he said, "I've been here for six years, I'm easy to get along with, and I know a lot of people."

A physician a generation older, a cardiologist in his fifties, described a similar checkered career, where his varied contacts allowed him to build up a specialty practice. He got his first job through a good friend who was also working for the same doctor he went to work for. He said:

> When I finished my house staff training, I went to work for a fellow who did vascular disease at the hospital, and I worked in his office for two years, and therefore developed an interest in vascular diseases. I saw his patients, was paid a salary, and also was given an opportunity to use his office when he was not there to see my own patients to build up my own practice. Then, probably five years after that, I was given the opportunity, untrained, to run the cardiac service at another affiliated hospital, because the guy that was there had some problems with the division, and he needed somebody who would kind of look after things. So he asked me if I would run the subdivision of cardiology, which I did. In that two or three years that I ran it, I read a lot of cardiology, I ran the conferences, and that sort of thing. That is really how I developed an interest in cardiology.

Women physicians are less likely to be offered opportunities to both build up their practices and to learn additional skills. An internist in her fifties stated that because she was a woman, she had been denied the chance to do physicals at a private clinic for executives that was located at her hospital when she was starting out. She said:

> Most of my male cohort received appointments in that clinic to examine executives of various companies. They were paid rather handsomely, and this was also very helpful in starting practice. Most of my male friends who did go into practice had this sort of little subsidy from the hospital. I was denied it. The reason they gave me was that there were no women executives who would want to get check-ups, and that men executives would object to being examined by a woman. I had asked both the director of the clinic and the chief of service, and both so very bluntly said, 'No, you cannot have it.' This was the most efficient way, and probably the most lucrative, at that time, for a physician to start a practice, and it was a prestigious place. Instead, I had to travel by subway to a telephone company downtown and spend three-quarters of an hour going there and back to examine the telephone company employees, which was nice in some ways, but it was certainly not as interesting as doing internist-type, comprehensive work-ups.

In the past, the kinds of positions women were referred to were jobs of lesser prestige – nursing homes, employee health services, and schools – where most of the patients are women or children, and few become private patients. Corporate-financed medicine will make more part-time positions available and these too may be relegated to women physicians (Starr 1982: 423). They will have little managerial control or prestige as salaried employees.

In early relationships with associates or partners, men operate as more or less autonomous equals; women are more often treated paternalistically. Three of the women physicans I interviewed, and one of the men, in fact went into practice with or shared offices with their fathers. A young woman dermatologist who originally shared an office with her father, an orthopedist, found that she was not learning how to run her own kind of practice. She met an established dermatologist at a professional meeting and went to his city to spend two weeks learning how he ran his practice thus hiring herself a mentor (M.P. Rowe 1977a). She said of her mentor:

> He helped me so much. He really taught me about handling patients and running a practice. It was an amazing experience. It made a real turning point in my life. As soon as I came back to my practice, it was easy – so easy.

Another woman dermatologist, now in her forties, described her helpful relationship with two physicians who were a great deal older than she:

> I began to work for those two doctors; I've been with them ever since. I went to work for them as a salaried person. They are both clinical professors and really through them, because I was really working for them, I had my entrance into the department. I didn't know anybody there.

In another case, the association seemed to have come about because the woman physician was the only one willing to put up with a disliked attending physician, and the relationship had overtones of exploitation for her. She said:

> He had a big practice, and he knew that I would be helpful to him, and we had personally gotten along. He knew I was a glutton for work, and I was not critical of him. A lot of people in the medical department sneered at him. I think he knew that I would be a friend to him, and I wouldn't get arrogant the way a lot of the other residents were about him. He knew that he was laughed at in the department, but I wasn't one who did it, so that

may be why I had some appeal to him. He allowed me the use of his office two afternoons a week. I simply was paid a straight salary from him plus being given use of all the office, which, of course, is equivalent to thousands of dollars of expense. I did an enormous amount of patient coverage. I covered for him alternating weekends and every night, plus taking care of my own practice. It was a monumental amount of work, but I did it for four years. I also learned a great deal from him as to how you run a practice.

We had no written contract. I laugh when I think about this. I know nothing about business, nothing. He asked me to come over before we could get this deal going, and I went over to his office, and he was sitting there with his lawyer and his accountant, and I come over in my little white coat from the wards and walk into this. I mean this was intimidating let me tell you.

She later went into a partnership practice with a man her own age she had trained with, who had had difficulties getting patients because he had inherited the practice of his antagonistic chief of service. It took him about three of four years before his hospital colleagues referred patients to him since, he said, "They thought I was fighting the same battle." In this case, too, the woman associate may have been giving more than she got back.

In the AAMC survey (see Appendix I), when medical students were asked to choose classmates they would most and least like as an office partner, women were much less likely to be preferred. Many women physicians of course do achieve thriving, and often well-paying, solo fee-for-service practices, and they have excellent relationships with colleagues in referrals of patients, consultations, and coverage arrangements. However, when their career development is compared, men have the advantage of lucrative or prestigious early opportunities, and are less likely to continue to work at salaried jobs (Bauder-Nishita 1980; Bobula 1980; Kutner and Brogan 1980; Wilson and A.B. Jones 1977; Kehrer 1976). This comparison, it should be noted, refers to *white* male and female physicians. Black physicians with office-based careers have many of the same problems as women physicians.

Getting patients:
"Ladies like to see ladies"?

Patients who choose physicians tend to prefer physicians of their own religion and ethnic background, and white patients in the United

States are very reluctant to consult black physicians, but women patients do not strongly or consistently prefer physicians of their own gender (Levinson, McCollum, and Kutner 1984; Ackerman-Ross and Sochat 1980). The issue of gender incongruity may be one of default. More women than men visit physicians, but since most physicians in the United States are men, unless women deliberately seek out women physicians, they are likely to be referred to male doctors. Since the physician is an authority figure and the patient often feels like a "passive object," it may go against the cultural grain for men to submit to women "for problems involving extensive handling, probing, and undressing," but not for women to submit to male physicians (Ackerman-Ross and Sochat 1980: 64). Expressed attitudes toward women physicians over the past thirty years have mostly been negative (Adams 1977; Engleman 1974; J.J. Williams 1950, 1946). A survey of 500 clinic patients found that "a significant percentage of the patients interviewed had never consulted a female physician yet did not hesitate to offer negative opinions of female physicians" (Engleman 1974: 99).

In the Soviet Union, where the majority of the physicians are women, male patients are routinely examined by women physicians. Like women patients in the United States, they have little choice but to consult physicians of the opposite sex. As women physicians become more numerous in the United States, women patients who prefer them will have more of a choice, and those who are neutral will have greater exposure to the experience. When the presence of women physicians is common, as it is getting to be on hospital house staffs and in clinics and group practices, patients with negative attitudes will be more reluctant to express them openly.

In a turnabout, one male physician I interviewed, a dermatologist, felt he was discriminated against because patients preferred to see one of his sisters, who was in practice in the same community. He said, "Ladies like to see ladies. There are even men who prefer to see lady doctors; they think they're more sympathetic." A woman general practitioner in her seventies similarly felt that "men go to women doctors when they are in trouble – for a mother image." However, a woman internist felt that men who sought out female physicians were "unsavory." She described two experiences with men who got her name from a hospital directory who she felt were psychosexually abnormal, and she now refuses any male patients who are not referred by someone she knows. Another internist felt she frequently got referrals of "crocks" or difficult patients because she was a woman and supposedly could handle these patients better than a male physician. In general, the gender composition of most of the practices of those interviewed depended on their specialty. Those with general practices had more women than men patients regardless of whether they themselves were male or female.

Relationships with patients:
"Appreciation for what we try to do"

Patients' choices of women or men physicians raises the perennial question of whether women doctors actually relate to patients differently from male physicians. Only one physician interviewed, a patient-oriented general practitioner, felt women and men physicians handled patients differently. She said, "Women in medicine by and large pay attention to small things. Most patients do not have major diseases – they have little annoying things. And also there's always a psychological component." Women physicians seem to relate better to dying patients, because they find it easier to tell the patient the bad news and to console families (Dickerson and Pearson 1979). Women physicians are sued for malpractice less frequently, which could be a function of their not being well-represented in the highest risk specialties of neurosurgery and orthopedics, or due to their more empathic or sympathetic relationships with their patients (Holder 1979). No physician can work competently without objectivity and some emotional self-protection (Daniels 1960; R.C. Fox 1957) so it may be that patients *perceive* women physicians to be attuned to feelings (Davidson 1975; see also Heins, Hendricks, and Martindale 1979). Also, women physicians may have an expressive behavior style. In actuality, women physicians and men physicians vary along the continuum from concern to detachment, with most following the well-known pattern of "detached concern."

To see whether, from the physicians' point of view, men and women relate to patients differently, I asked what kinds of patients they liked most and least. The responses from the male and female physicians in office-based practice were monotonously similar. From the women, best liked patients were "young, basically healthy, pleasant, and easy to get along with," "cooperative," "successful, self-assured, interested in knowing," "intelligent," "normal, straight-forward," "very educated and very achieved." From the men, best liked were patients who are "medically compliant, understanding, well-paying," "appreciate what you're trying to do," "middle-class, moderately educated," "my kind, my level of education, easy to get on with and don't question your expertise," "a person where there's some kind of intervention that can help," "bright, successful, creative."

Male and female physicians were equally similar in their descriptions of the patients they liked least. The women disliked patients who were "demanding," "had chronic pain," "lunatic of the month," "worry-wort, completely dissatisfied," "neurotic and demanding," "narciss-istic," "very garrulous, very demanding, very manipulative," "tells you what to do." The men disliked patients who were "nit-picking," "show an obvious suspicion, lack of confidence from the outset, hostile and aggressive," "question without good reason," "argue with you about every medical decision," "call up several times a day, about minor problems."

In short, women and men physicians, like most medical workers, prefer patients who allow them to carry out their tasks with a minimum of fuss, make little trouble, and are cooperative, trusting, and appreciative of their care, and are likely to benefit from their treatment. Problem patients for both male and female physicians are those with intractable physical problems, who complain a great deal, are very emotional, anxious, need a lot of reassurance, encouragement, and attention. They are especially disliked when they are not very sick (Lorber 1975b). Although many patients come to doctors' offices with minor complaints and just need someone to talk to, physicians are trained to deal with serious illnesses and life-threatening pathologies, and they often consider many of their consultations to be "trivial, unnecessary, or inappropriate" (A. Cartwright and Anderson 1981). There is little indication that women physicians are more feeling-oriented than their male colleagues, and patients who seek sympathy from them and do not get it may turn hostile.

The similarity of attitudes of women and men physicians to patients may be the result of the selection of medical students who are good in science rather than in interpersonal relationships and the heavily scientific and objectified medical education they undergo. The need to see many patients to earn more money or to manage an extensive pre-paid practice workload also tends to restrict involvement, as does the routinization of response that occurs to most people in service occupations.

Joining the colleague community:
"There's a club there"

Since physicians in office practice are heavily dependent on their colleagues for referrals of patients, they are more likely to get referrals if they are part of a colleague community, either as a member of an "inner circle" or as a friendly familiar face. For physicians in the United States today, the hospital is the locus of the colleague community, and it is very important to have an affiliation at a hospital where one is visible and accepted. In addition, office-based physicians need hospital affiliations in order to admit their patients and continue to see them, and they must be extended the courtesy of visiting privileges by other physicians, full or part-time, on the hospital's staff. Finally, the hospital is the place to see more varied medical problems through the care of clinic patients, and to keep up with the latest medical procedures through case conferences and grand rounds. Those office-based physicians who are affiliated with a teaching hospital also have a chance to do clinical teaching to interns and residents in their own rounds of their patients' bedsides.

Generally, visiting privileges at a hospital are extended to office-based physicians who trained there as house staff or fellows. They have already worked with the physicians on the staff in caring for their hospitalized patients, and in house-call coverage over nights and weekends. Unless the hospital has a policy of only allowing full-time staff members to admit patients, most office-based physicians get "privileges" where they trained.

The difficulty of establishing a hospital base when one is not known is well illustrated by an endocrinologist in her thirties who was denied a full-time position at the hospital where she had done her most recent training, and where she had had no trouble getting referrals. She was trying to work into the colleague community at another hospital in the city, where she had done her earlier training, and where she was not as well known. Since she was not as comfortable there as she was at her current hospital affiliation, she felt she wasn't putting in all the effort she should to break into "the club." In her own words:

> I'm out of the mainstream there. I come to make rounds and I go back up here. There's a club there. A club of members, where you would have coffee together, and you would be out there politicking, bullshitting, and talking, and wasting a lot of time, and getting the referrals. I don't do any of that there, so I don't get any consults there. Here, I'm visible enough. I trained here, I stayed on here, I make rounds, people see me, and I don't have to go through all of that. There, I would have to. I did my internship and residency there, but the couple of years makes the difference. They want you loyal. They don't like hearing about you going back and forth. It's a very ingrained place.

Her problems are those of any stranger trying to break into an established community. Still, gender congruity can make it easier. Some of the older women who trained at the medical center where the interviews were done were steered to an affiliated women's hospital, now closed, at the start of their careers. The entire academic staff of this hospital – the heads of departments, teaching physicians, and residents – were women. There were consultants and courtesy staff who were male, but the full-time staff was all female. One physician who was on the staff described what it was like:

> I think there was a special quality at the hospital. There was a lot of pride among the women and respect for the tradition because it had been exceedingly hard for women to become physicians.

The contrast in ambience in a male-dominated hospital is summed up by the following anecdote from a hematologist in her forties. She said:

> I went to witness a Caesarian section of a hematology patient. The chief resident was a woman. Most of the people in the delivery room at that point were women. When I went to change, there wasn't any place to change at all. They just ignored the fact that perhaps the women would need someplace to put on their scrub suits. There was one very small women's bathroom. The chief resident had already hung her clothes on the one hook, so I hung up my clothes on the hook over her clothes, and hoped that they wouldn't fall off. There is no women's changing room on the surgical floor. There is no lounge for women in this entire medical center.

For the most part, integration into a colleague community for women physicians is getting easier. At one time, a woman who practiced in a small town was totally isolated. Now in her fifties, one recalled:

> I was the only woman doctor in the community. I had no peers and I was ostracized and shunned by the men I worked with, and I was ostracized and shunned by the women of the community because I was different.

Another woman in her fifties who had worked in a nursing home was also ignored by her male colleagues:

> When people would go to lunch, they wouldn't say to you, "Are you coming?" It wouldn't occur to them. Most of those men had

taken their internships together; they had all known each other for a great many years; they were all in private practice on the outside and I was not; I was a good deal older than they; my kids were a lot older.

However, later, when two other women physicians came, who had common interests with her, they did not form a group:

Our tendency was not to sit around and palsy walsy when you got the work done. There were other things waiting to be done at home. From long practice, you just finished one job and went to the other, because nobody was going to do it at home. Whereas the guys – all they had to do was go home for dinner. It was different and legitimately so. I never felt resentful of it.

Younger women physicians, even when married, are better integrated into colleague networks. A woman dermatologist in her forties with four children has lunch once a week with the members of her department, of whom several are women. They also include residents, to whom she acts as a kind of role model. Of them she said, "A lot of them are married and have children, and they're very anxious about that. They want to speak to you about how you manage." Another woman in her forties said of her colleagues, "We have a very close department. Really very good friends. It is certainly one of the warmest, closest relationships that anybody could ever want. Really very supportive."

Men of all ages can still be found in close-knit, all male colleague networks. A dermatologist in his fifties was a member of two all male dermatologic societies of about twenty to twenty-five doctors who met once a month to present patients and discuss cases, and have hors d'oeuvres and cocktails and sit around and talk. Of the lack of women, he said:

There's nothing in the constitution that would not allow woman members. I, for one, have proposed women for membership and haven't gotten anywhere, not because of the members, but because the proposed women simply had other things to do with their time. They are either raising a family or they don't have time to go to meetings and countless other things.

But he admitted not having looked around for women who might have the time, nor did he suggest altering the time of the meetings occasionally to fit a married woman's schedule.

Women themselves frequently do not see the worth of professional socializing. By not defining these activities as an intrinsic part of their work life, women, unlike men, do not assign them a high priority. Thus, in a dual-career marriage, it is the husband, rather than the wife, who is likely to engage in professional social activities, meetings, and conferences. The wife, particularly if there are children, is more likely to give her family duties a higher priority than the social part of her professional life.

Even non-professional socializing, when it involves colleagues, tends to revolve around the men's friends, and to include the wives only as wives (Lipman-Blumen 1976). Two men described such social networks as all male by default of the small numbers of women in medicine. A forty-year-old oncologist said of his group of male colleagues and their wives:

> These are surgeons that I work with at the hospital and they happen to be male surgeons. They're not being picked because they're male or female; they're picked because they are people I work with and am friendly with. We found that whenever we happen to be at the same meetings we enjoy being together and not just talking shop but talking anything, and we found we were just not meeting frequently enough so we decided to make it a regular thing. We now meet once a month and have dinner together with our wives someplace.

A cardiologist in his thirties, a bachelor, had a social-professional network of cardiologists who were competitive and not in a referral network, but still friends. When asked why there were no women in the group, he said it was because there were no women cardiologists when he was trained. Nonetheless, even among male physicians who trained or worked with women, many social-professional networks are all male (and all white).

Even the best-integrated women can have difficulties with their colleagues, whose status expectations of them still relegates them to secondary places. A woman dermatologist in her fifties was asked if she minded being passed over in favor of her brother as head of the dermatology service at the suburban hospital where she was affiliated. She said:

> I do give a hoot about titles and I'm enough of a feminist not to let them promote my brother over me. I have put in many years more of service, and I'm a far better dermatologist than my brother. They tried to do this to me because I'm a woman.

Those, excuse the French, assholes, said to me, "Do you mind us promoting your brother over you? He needs the honor." And I said, "For the sake of the women who follow after me, I mind. I do not accept that explanation." And they said, "Well if you come to our meetings, we can't tell dirty jokes, and we can't take off our shoes." I said, "Bull to that one. I know just as many dirty jokes as you do, and I always take off my shoes." All the board of trustees laughed like hell when they heard about it. They all said, "For god's sake, promote her." Most of them were patients of mine anyway. It's a stupid thing to say to a woman doctor. I don't care for me, but I want to make sure that the next generation gets a fair shake and doesn't get it in the eye.

She was promoted and became the first woman full attending and the first woman chief of service at that hospital.

Women's colleague networks:
"Who needs them?"

Using Hall's continuum of physicians as members of an inner circle, friendly colleagues, and isolates, I would argue that most women with office-based careers are friendly colleagues or isolates, although there are a few who are members of an inner circle. Only one of the women physicians interviewed was trying to build up a female colleague referral network. This internist, now in her fifties, said, "Whenever possible, and whenever the specificities are good, I would prefer to send many of my patients to a woman." Ironically, a colleague network homogeneous on gender is still likely to exclude on other social characteristics. A woman in her thirties who described herself as flirtatious and feminine, and who was having a hard time getting referrals, said she knew she should become friendlier with the women gynecologists, but, she said, "All the women gynecologists in this city are militant feminists. Who needs them? Those women who go to a woman militant do not want to come to me." Nonetheless, where there are sufficient numbers of women physicians, colleague referrals are one of the easiest ways to create female professional networks, since they are under the control of the individual physician.

While there may not be enough senior women in any one medical institution or community to form a referral network, local, regional, and national women's medical organizations serve as a source of contacts, information exchange, and support (Lewin 1982; Harlin

1981; Scadron 1980; Yokopenic, Bourque, and Brogan 1975). These women's medical organizations allow women physicians to form their own inner circle whose numbers can give them significant leverage in their home institutions and in male-dominated professional organizations. There does not have to be a choice between male and female colleague networks – many physicians belong to more than one professional group, such as general medical associations and various specialty associations – and identify themselves with more than one set of colleagues. Indeed, identification with a group of women physicians can give an individual physician the visibility she needs to become part of the male establishment. However, unless the women's groups maintain their strength and separate identity, the integration of a few women into male-dominated inner circles is not likely to change conditions in such a way as to make it possible for all women physicians who so desire to talk shop over lunch, go out to dinner, tell dirty jokes, and be promoted to full attending and chief of service.

Chapter 5
CAREERS IN ACADEMIC MEDICINE:
getting ahead

"The medical school would never support my being
chief of service"
(Woman physician)

Physicians in the United States with careers in academic medicine do
clinical research, see patients as part of a faculty or part-time private
practice, and teach in medical schools. Part of their income comes
from research grants and part is salary from the hospital and medical
school. This base salary is often supplemented by a percentage of the
fees brought in by the patients they care for, and by lectures, books, or
other outside work. Careers in academic medicine may pay less than
office-based practices, but the physician has the advantages of office
and laboratory space, secretarial and technical personnel, a guaran-
teed income, and a regular time schedule. As one male respondent
said of such a career:

> The advantage of academic medicine is the variety. One does not
> sit and see patients every day. Teaching and interaction with
> students are intellectually stimulating and fun. The research is
> enjoyable. You do not have to feel incumbent to be on call every
> few minutes, and you have some time for your family.

A career in academic medicine may be attractive to research-
oriented women physicians, but full-time appointments at prestigious
teaching hospitals and medical schools are not easily come by.[1]
Getting the first position is a hurdle, and, as in other professional
careers, help from sponsors is extremely valuable (Epstein 1970a). A

clinical investigator, like other scientists, must obtain financial support for research or work with someone who has ongoing projects. Here, too, senior people can be very helpful (Reskin 1978a; Zuckerman 1978).

Career advancement depends on expanding research production, publishing, getting referrals of patients for clinical research, and obtaining more autonomy by becoming director of a laboratory, a hospital unit, or an entire service. As careers in academic medicine develop, the recognition and support of colleagues who are at the same level is necessary for invitations to present papers and give lectures, for citations to one's work, for promotion, and for referrals. For those who, in addition, want to build up a private practice, referrals are essential.

Women are more likely to be sponsored during their training period and men during their actual career development. While women are acceptable as heads of small units and may run their own laboratories, they are unlikely to be promoted to upper level positions in hospitals and medical schools (Farrell, *et al.* 1979). Although the women I interviewed had productive careers and some were internationally known researchers, the most prestigious position held by a woman over the age of fifty was temporary chief of a department of internal medicine. In contrast, six of the eight men interviewed who were over fifty were or had been chiefs of departments or services, and one had also been head of a hospital.

Getting the first position: "Knowing the right people"

In medicine, residencies and fellowships not only provide intensive training in a specialty, but also allow senior physicians to observe the quality of junior physicians' performances as clinicians and researchers. This assessment by established physicians sorts the novices into potential colleagues and those who are encouraged to go elsewhere. The hallmark of this informal sorting process is first-hand knowledge of the young physician, who must not only perform in a way that is acceptable to his or her future colleagues, but must also be visible to them. The intensely personalized nature of the process encourages young physicians to seek appointments where they have trained and are known. As an oncologist in his thirties described it, "I was here already, and the chief of service said, 'Do you want to come on the staff?'" A female specialist in pulmonary disorders, also in her thirties, had an open invitation to return to the institution where she had been a resident. She said:

> When I was resident, I came here and did a rotation in infectious diseases, and Dr –, who was head of the department and a very influential man, knew I was going into pulmonary medicine and said, "Please, when you're finished with your fellowship, come back. We need somebody desperately in pulmonary medicine." So, because I had been here, and enjoyed it, and it was certainly very challenging, I thought it would be nice to come back.

Alternatively, when new physicians seek a position in a hospital or research institute where they have not trained, they usually depend very heavily on the personal recommendation of someone who knows them.[2] The personalized quality of the search for jobs in medical academia is summed up in the following comment by a young male hematologist:

> I didn't know there was a position available. I knew who was the chief. I knew that my chief was very friendly with the chief here, so that it would not be a difficult problem to come here. They both knew each other very well, and so part of it was my application, and part of it was knowing the right people. That's not a strange way of getting a position.

In the early stages, women and men physicians who want careers in academic medicine are equally likely to be recognized and supported for junior faculty positions. Women who are in the later stages of their careers, however, report difficulty sustaining their early advances.

Career advancement:
"He had heard of me"

Women in male-dominated settings need an extra boost if their achievements are to be taken seriously and if they are to be considered for leadership positions. In experiments with mixed-sex small task groups, the status of the women is enhanced by planting "information" that they are especially expert in the task the group is to accomplish, or by simply appointing a woman as leader of the group (Fennell *et al.* 1978; Meeker and Weitzel-O'Neill 1977; Eskilon and Wiley 1976; Lockheed and K.P. Hall 1976). In real life, the devalued status of women can be counteracted by the timely support of powerful sponsors who can help establish credibility, competence, and trustworthiness as colleagues.

A sponsor or patron ("godfather" or "rabbi" are other terms frequently used) is a crucial part of the advancement process for any physician, because it is sponsors who suggest opportunities, facilitate promotions, and act as go-betweens in negotiations. While sponsors take men under their wing routinely, women usually have to bring themselves to a sponsor's attention if they want to advance. There are three methods of getting attention for women physicians – lucky breaks, extraordinary accomplishments, and self-presentation. They counteract the general invisibility of women who are not routinely rewarded for good work performance.

THE LUCKY BREAK

One woman, in her fifties when interviewed, recalled how she was given a break that overcame the two strikes against her – being a woman and being the graduate of a foreign medical school.[3] Of her initial opportunity, she said:

> I went to a very prestigious hospital for an interview and was accepted to my great surprise. I was the only foreign graduate and I was the first woman resident in that particular service. The interviewer was trained by a very famous Hungarian physician. During the interview, the interviewer recalled his experience with this physician. He said one of the reasons why he'd give me a chance is because I'm Hungarian. It was political chic at that time, too, to have Hungarian physicians. I don't give myself special credit – my English was bad and I don't think my training was so outstanding. Being Hungarian was probably the main thing.

She was able to expand this excellent residency into a fellowship and then a staff appointment, because, she felt, she was "very good."

Another woman foreign medical graduate now in her forties recalled how she got her accidental start in a subspecialty of hematology that made her a well-known "grandmother" in the field:

> Before I became an attending here I was a fellow, and every Monday morning I used to have a cup of coffee with the chief of the service. Just having a cup of coffee, he asked me, "Would you like a machine – a new kind of machine? All I know is that it

separates blood," I said, "Why not?" And that is how the whole story started. About three weeks later I get a call that the machine is here, and from a one-person operation I have now five machines – the other applications for this machine I pioneered.

In these two cases, the sponsor offered entrée into a good training institution or access to new technology, but it was the women's own subsequent efforts that advanced their careers. Without the initial sponsorship, however, they would not have been in a position where they could demonstrate their abilities. In the opposite situation, where abilities are already evident, recognition by a sponsor can help a woman achieve the next stage in her career development, but does not necessarily smooth the way to a steady climb.

EXTRAORDINARY ACCOMPLISHMENT

Devalued social characteristics can be overridden by extraordinary accomplishments which single out the person as someone special and not to be measured by the usual expectations for his or her group. Their careers are dependent on the continued support of sponsors who help them advance, but the sponsors may limit their autonomy or isolate them from other women (Reskin 1978a; Kanter 1977b; Laws 1975; Epstein 1974b, 1970a). The following account illustrates both the benefits and costs of sponsorship dependent on extraordinary accomplishment.

A clinical researcher throughout her career, a woman physician in her forties had published seven papers in her junior year as a medical student. Her unusual abilities brought her to the attention of a professor in a prominent research institute that was part of the medical center where she was an intern. In her words:

When I was an intern, Dr –, who was a professor at the research institute, heard about me and called me up and asked me if I wanted to join his staff when I finished. I said I wanted to do a first-year residency, so he held the position for me. I went from being a resident one day to being assistant professor with my own laboratory the next day. I had never met Dr – before, but he had heard about me, and knew about my background. So I went over and joined his group. I never asked Dr – specifically why he identified me. He seemed to know all about what I had done. I published papers in one of the institute's journals and I think that Dr – read them, and then happened to be someplace where publicly he mentioned it, and someone said, "You know, she's just across the street as an intern." He ran his department with a great deal of flexibility, so he identified people, and asked them to come, and if they worked out, and the field blossomed, they stayed.

Her field blossomed to the point where it became a subspecialty in internal medicine with separate laboratories in almost every major medical institution, except her own. She spent ten years as part of her sponsor's laboratory group. They got grants and published papers together, with equal authorship, and she followed him when he went to another part of the medical center. By the time he left, her work was autonomous enough so that she was not affected by his leaving, but she did not get her own laboratory space until the medical center was under affirmative action pressure. She said:

My opportunity was made because the dean and the chair of the department of medicine were reviewing people within the department. At the time, I guess they were seeing what women were doing, and what men were doing, and where they were going and I guess they just came up with this space which was available, and I was the logical person to begin with. I think I got it because of my published work, and that I had created a new field and the dean realized it was what I had done and my collaborator was the first to admit that I had essentially done it. There was a laboratory for this work in every medical school in the country. Looking it over, this was the logical step to do – to set one up here. So I was given this space. They were just grubby old labs, and they didn't have any ceilings or anything. It was being given to me to do whatever I wanted to do, my own time, and at that time I had enough support to make up the staff, so I could be independent. They were very nice financially. I could take all the equipment that I had accumulated, and the department and the university contributed to my salary, so it was a very salubrious relationship. I think everybody who is in academic medicine who has developed something as I had, wants eventually to stand on their own two feet.

Although she was a recognized international authority with many publications and an established grant recipient with a staff she supported, when her sponsor left, she never thought to insist on her own laboratory space or on physical accommodations commensurate with her accomplishments, nor did her former sponsor or the dean or the chair of the department feel she should be so rewarded.

SELF-PRESENTATION

Younger women physicians seem to be more aware of what they may be entitled to. The reverse of the older physician encouraging the younger was described to me by a nephrologist in her fifties. She said of her younger colleague:

> She is much more gung ho about these things than I am and has pushed. She says that if I'd pushed earlier, she wouldn't have to push so hard now. Since I am ahead of her in time, she feels that she can't get anything until I've gotten it, so she's pushing me.

Young women are also more willing to go to a powerful person and present their credentials and accomplishments if they feel they are not being adequately rewarded. Self-presentation to a potential sponsor requires having confidence in past performance and clear goals for future work. It sometimes means bypassing an immediate superior and going directly to the most powerful and influential person in the work situation. When faced with organizational politics, the ability and willingness to leapfrog to the most powerful sponsors one can approach is an extremely valuable asset. This technique of professional advancement has long been used by men.

A male physician in his forties used it successfully twice in his career. While this physician was still in training, he had arranged to join a group working on kidney transplants on his return from a two-year fellowship abroad. By the time he returned, the head of the group had moved into the department of surgery. He felt that his position there would not be good for his career. In his words:

> Although my professional work was quite adequate – quite good – politically as a very junior member of the staff, I had no future in the department of surgery. There was a lot of competition – for space, for bodies. Through my wife, who was firmly rooted in Medicine – remember, I was outside of Medicine – the chairman of the department got to know me and he said, "You know, you're doing such good work, the surgeons don't understand you, that's not a very good group, so why don't you join Medicine."

A year and a half later he did join the department of internal medicine, and under the chair, a rival nephrology group was set up. Unfortunately, the group that had been in surgery eventually came back to the department of internal medicine, and the chair of the department left, so this doctor was again out in the cold. He got another powerful sponsor, the new head of a different hospital and research institute in the medical center, a doctor who was a specialist in a related field. In describing his new sponsor, the nephrologist said:

> I would probably have left, but Dr – offered me the job of director of kidney diseases over there. It seemed like a reasonable opportunity, obviously. He is world famous, and he also made it very attractive.

After that, this physician was able to generate his own funding for research, and then he went on to obtain an endowed professorship in a totally different field.

Deliberate self-presentation to people in a position to advance one's career is a very useful strategy, but it calls for assurance, contacts in high places, and the realization that merit is not necessarily its own reward. Women physicians whose professional development coincided with the burgeoning women's movement are willing to play this game (Romm 1982).

Two female clinical researchers in their thirties described how they had bypassed their immediate superiors to get the support of more powerful sponsors. Looking for her first position after training, one of them was offered jobs in cities in which she did not want to live. In her own institution, the head of her unit was not interested in offering her a staff position. She went to the director of the institute where she was a fellow and where she wanted to stay. She said he had "sort of taken me under his wing." She told him about the job offers and tactfully asked his advice as to whether it would be a good idea for her professionally to take one of these jobs:

> And he said, "Why are you leaving?" And I said, "I didn't know I had any alternatives." He said, "You shouldn't leave." And I said, "Well, who's going to pay me? I'm not willing to be a fellow anymore." He said, "No, of course not." The next thing I knew I had a job.

Another clinical researcher was being exploited by her boss, who insisted on having his name on her papers and research proposals, and who would not put her up for assistant professor despite (or perhaps because of) the success of a new program for diabetic mothers she had started. She went job hunting, and had three offers to come with her new program:

> With that in my back pocket, I went to the department of medicine chairman and asked him to hire me as *his* faculty member and assistant professor and at a good salary. And he gave it to me. It took about a year.

71

Both of these women were young, and the men they sought out to intervene for them were powerful, senior physicians. As they advance, they will have to deal with male colleagues who are their peers or only one step above them. The question, then, is whether their bids to advance will be honored.

Getting to the top:
"A woman of aspirations"

As in other academic careers, physicians in academic medicine seek promotion and tenure. Publications, presentations at meetings, and reputations in one's field are the counters used by status evaluators and gatekeepers along the upward climb. These markers count for less, though, when women are involved. Three cases illustrate the contrast between men and women in getting to the top.

In the first case, a highly productive and successful researcher in her forties discussed the possible constraints on her career advancement. She was at a prestigious research and teaching institution which had never had a woman full professor. She said:

> I'm the only woman who's never been head of a lab – but I'm not tenured. This is a long-term question for me. I have had offers for tenured full professor slots – but at places not of the caliber that I've been accustomed to. It's been an unusual thing, these offers – and one was at triple my salary. They are for full professor and head of a division, department or special hospital unit. In one place, the problems were two-fold – the intellectual environment, and secondly, a huge administrative load. If you look at the top prestige places, there are very few women professors of academic medicine. I don't dwell on it. I am extraordinarily fortunate – I have been able to get my grants, I have had a good group of people working for me, I'm working in an exciting area, and I have fantastic collaborators. So I am very lucky – but I am a woman of aspirations, so I can't tell you that I wouldn't like it to go further.

The kind of offers she is getting indicate that extremely well-qualified women will be able to get to the top – but not necessarily in the most highly regarded institutions.

The career of the woman who had achieved the most prestigious position of all the women interviewed, acting head of a large department of internal medicine, illustrates the difficulty women still face in trying to break the invisible barrier to the highest positions in the medical world. She was in her fifties when she was interviewed.

Her first job was in a chronic disease institution, where she did patient care and clinical research as head of a division. After five years, the director of the medical service became head of the department of internal medicine at a well-regarded general hospital, and asked her to go with him as his assistant. Subsequently, she was made an associate professor. During her sponsor's sabbatical, she ran the department as acting director. She continued to do research, publish, and give presentations at national and international meetings. Yet, when her sponsor was about to retire, she was not put on the list for possible chief of services by the search committee.

When she realized she would not even be considered for a position she had already shown she could handle, she left the hospital and went into private practice, sharing an office with her husband, who was in a different specialty. He was affiliated with another medical center, and she was given a courtesy affiliation. She had no laboratory space, no research patients, and was cut off entirely from her former colleague community. This is her story in her own words:

> My chief, whom I worked for for thirteen years, was about to retire. He's an older man. I was not considered to be the successor. I didn't feel I got a fair shake. I thought I should have been the next chief. If I tell you it was because I am a woman, that's a very simple statement, although I think that had a great deal to do with it. I ran that service pretty independently when my chief was on sabbatical. I think I did a very good job. I was named acting chief. They never even told me they would not consider me. I just put out feelers. I put in a request for promotion to full professor. I had twenty-eight papers and foreign presentations. I ran the service independently for several months. The medical school sent back my promotion request saying that my contributions are strong, but not internationally strong enough to make me a full professor. That really made me furious because many of my fellow professors were everything but internationally strong enough to be full professors. I thought that was really the indication that the medical school would never support my being the chief of that service. It's a pretty big service – about one hundred and fifty attendings and seventy house staff.

Her productivity and reputation may not have been great enough to guarantee being named permanent chief of one of the most prestigious services in a medical center, but combined with her previous experience in the position, they should at least have qualified her for consideration by the search committee.

The contrast with males is well illustrated by the smooth history of a male cardiologist, also in his fifties, who described the time-honored way he built his career through the sponsorship of established physicians. He said:

> I went into practice at the medical center. It was what we call geographical full-time, where two or three days a week I would see my private patients in this little part-time office which was set up for private practice and lab testing, and the rest of the time, I was up in cardiology continuing my research project. I got patients because in my young time I was often asked to help and take calls at night and weekends and vacations for some leading practitioners. One quite famous practitioner often sent me a patient for consultation or evaluation, and I got to know a lot of his patients. The doctor I'd worked with for my fellowship had a very, very plush cardiology practice, and I was his assistant. The head of the department of medicine would send me patients because he wouldn't see private patients very often. There was a community of doctors there, like it always happens in medical centers. I began to get more referrals than I could handle.

He eventually became head of his division, full professor, and then director of a prestigious hospital in the same medical center, taking his place in the succession of leaders of this community of doctors. He did not need a lucky break or especially extraordinary accomplishments in his rise. Later on, when he wanted to move to another medical center, he played the reluctant "bride" in what he described a two-year courtship in which he steadily upped his ante, letting an intermediary successfully present his credentials, plans, and demands to the institution. He moved as a head of a unit located in beautifully renovated offices, and was named to an endowed full professorship.

In the high-powered, politicized world of prestigious medical centers, there is no doubt that the ability to "hustle" is an asset for a successful career. This is not to say that a non-hustler will not do good work or make wonderful contributions to the conquering of disease and to the care of patients. It is the difference between, as one male physician put it, being a national or international authority in one's field, and being known only in the local medical community. The key to the visibility, he felt, was to make early political connections that facilitate later professional accomplishments. In his words:

> If there was one thing in my career I would do over, I would go a route where I made more political connections. I would also be a little bit more social. I sort of succeeded in a way. But it might have helped in the sense that those people who make major contributions frequently have students who make major contributions, so had I been a protégé of somebody who was very stimulating, I might have been stimulated to do something. I never had someone like that along the way to act as my mentor. The second way is in the political sense that it might have been helpful, but that might have been hard to document because I don't know where I could have gotten. I think just in terms of being called on more often as the authority in this field, I guess is really what it amounts to.

The political aspect of career advancement is a game of reciprocity. Sponsors support protégés, and protégés do work to which the sponsor's name is also attached as a joint author or in citations. Sponsors recommended protégés for committee chairs and session organizers at professional meetings. The up-and-coming physician can then invite the sponsor and other powerful and better known physicians to participate. For each, the circle of colleagues is widened. Invitees reciprocate by inviting; the lesser known gain visibility, and careers advance (H. Zuckerman 1977; Merton 1968).

Women can lose out in two ways. First, they may not be assertive enough in presenting themselves and their worth to potential sponsors. Here, we have seen, younger women seem less reluctant to put themselves forward. But their bids must be accepted, their worth must be given due credit, and they need someone to start them in the game of professional reciprocity. There are still pockets of negative attitudes towards women among some men who are in positions to recruit women and further their careers. One man, a very powerful cardiologist who was on many search and promotion committees, said:

> I don't think women ever had a bad deal, and I think this women's lib thing is overrated. A woman could always get into medical school, it seems to me. Very few of them applied when I was a kid, and not many women wanted to be a doctor compared to men. I don't think there was an exclusion. In fact it was easy, in my class, or that era, for women to get in with lower ranks than

75

men, and men had to compete against a lot more men. With five or six women in the class, they were often not very distinguished in their cerebral power, because it wasn't so hard for a woman to become a doctor. Nobody wanted to. I don't think women have ever been picked on. I think people like to make a case for it, but I don't see it.

He had one woman physician working part-time in his current unit. She had graduated first in her class from a prestigious medical school in 1950.

A second physician, an endocrinologist and head of a department half of whom were women, had this to say when asked about his knowledge of sex discrimination:

I took all comers as they came, and it just so happened at the time there were positions, those women were the most qualified, so I took them. I don't have certain attitudes which other physicians have about women on the service. I think that some of my colleagues feel that some of the women don't really carry their weight as much as some of the men do, that they would have outside obligations which would interfere with them doing their job completely. I don't really believe that at all. It's turned out that my own experience has never been that. So it comes out that it's not so much that I have done anything active to recruit women. I think others are doing something in their recruiting that in effect disqualifies women.

Between these two extremes of positive and negative attitudes toward women physicians, with their self-fulfilling effect, lie the feelings of most male physicians. They profess neutrality or good intentions, but do not actively recruit or support women. For that matter, women physicians who were high enough placed to promote other women do not do so either, because they feel uncomfortable about focussing on social characteristics as well as on merit.

Many women physicians, as we have seen, were given support during their careers, but few, if any, were thought of by their male colleagues as potential chairs of prestigious departments or as heads of major hospitals or research institutes. Many of these women had raised substantial governmental and philanthropic financing for their work; they ran laboratories, special programs, and hospital units; they published extensively; they gave papers at national and international professional meetings; and some were even pioneers in their fields. None the less, just as in Frank and Katcher's study of

medical students (Frank and Katcher 1977) their male peers seemed
unable to perceive them as leaders.

Women in medical academia:
"A handful in the whole department"

Whatever the hidden processes, the result is that there are currently
few women in leadership positions in medical academia in the United
States (Braslow and Heins 1981; Farrell *et al.* 1979). The authors of
one study comment:

> The data confirm the general impression that within the
> leadership of the vast majority of medical schools, women
> physicians are indeed hard to find. They are clustered in low,
> characteristically untenured faculty positions, largely in the
> traditional nurturant specialties or primarily in administrative
> posts that deal exclusively with student and minority affairs.
> Many medical schools as well as numerous individual depart-
> ments have no women physicians either at the professor or
> associate professor level or in any administrative post.
>
> (Farrell *et al.* 1979: 2810–811)

How such a situation feels to a woman in medical academia was
described by one of the physicians interviewed, an associate professor
in her forties. She said:

> There is one other woman who is a member of the senior faculty
> staff in this division. There are a handful in the whole
> department. I try to count the women at faculty meetings
> sometimes – there are never more than ten.

Data from four medical schools located in different parts of the
United States showed that it tended to take twice as long for women as
for men to go up the ladder from assistant to associate to full professor
(Wallis, Gilder and Thaler 1981). Even in the department of
pediatrics of a northeastern medical school, which was considered to
be "the most liberal and woman-accepting department," there was a
promotion lag for women. This study used as a comparative indicator
only years of service, and did not compare contributions of men and
women in research, publications, teaching, care of patients, and
administration, but the authors comment that *all* the women who had
gone through medical school in three decades could not have shown so

little productivity as to warrant the "blatant inequities" in promotion rates. In their words:

> It is hard to accept the implication that the same women physician graduates of the 1940s, 1950s, and 1960s, who passed through the bottleneck of medical college admissions, residency training, and faculty acceptance, deteriorated sufficiently in the quality of their contribution in the 1960s and 1970s so as to warrant the discrepancy in the promotion rates documented in this study. (Wallis, Gilder, and Thaler 1981: 2352).

The contributions of women are simply not given the same weight as those of men (White 1981). A nephrologist in her forties described how she had to bring her work to the attention of her boss to get promoted from assistant to associate professor. As she described it:

> I began to complain loudly. I went to the department chairman and said, "Here's what I'm working on." He said, "Well, everybody does that." My answer was, "Everybody else has been promoted to associate attending and associate professor, but I have not." Well, lo and behold, six months later, I got promoted!

Does it make a difference whether or not women physicians are in a position to influence research and curriculum development and the attitudes of medical students towards patients and the delivery of health care? (Relman 1980; Beuf 1978; Bluestone 1978; Howell 1974) Students, male and female, who are sensitive to patients' needs, are hardened by an education dominated by an emphasis on efficiency, rationality, and objectivity. Whatever might be different about women when they enter medical school, they are often indistinguishable from male physicians in their values and orientations when they graduate (Leserman 1981; Ginzberg 1978; Levitt 1977; Ortiz 1975). One study of women and men medical students found that although the women came in with humanitarian and politically liberal attitudes, both women and men left with a conservative outlook on patient care and medical system reforms, suggesting that the prevailing attitudes of the schools were more compatible with the men's views (Leserman 1981).

Women physicians have started to change medical school curricula and views on patient–doctor interaction.[4] So far, though, they have had little effect on the overall structure of medical institutions. Mary Howell, a feminist physician, has suggested separate medical schools and hospitals run by and for women, a throwback to the nine-teenth century (Howell 1975). Such separatism in the twentieth century would defeat the goal of integration of women into the medical establishment, and also deprive male patients and male colleagues of the benefit of women physicians' ideas about profession-al work. Whether or not women physicians do offer a different perspective, any effective physician, male or female, should have a chance to guide the medical profession if we are to have the best available medical services.

Notes

1 The percentage of women physicians in the United States who are full-time hospital staff is larger than that of men physicians, according to the American Medical Association's 1980 *Profile of Medical Practice* (Wunderman 1980), but many of these positions are in non-teaching hospitals, such as clinical staff of Veteran's Administration hospitals, and radiologists, anesthetists, emergency room physicians, etc. in community hospitals. The percentage of women and men in teaching, administration, and research is about the same: 2–3 per cent (Wunderman 1980). For an analysis of the current situation of academic physicians, see "Symposium on the Academic Physician: An Endangered Species," 1981.

2 On the "seeding" process in academic medicine, see S.J. Miller 1970.

3 On the relative status of foreign medical school graduates and women, see Goldblatt and Goldblatt 1976.

4 See Wallis, Gilder, and Thaler, 1981; Hubbard 1977. Dr Wallis is the organizer of the Cornell University Medical College Teaching Associates Program and the Tristate Regional Teaching Associates Network, which trains teaching associates to teach medical students and licensed physicians how to do breast, pelvic, and rectal examinations with sensitivity to patients' feelings. The March 1984 issue of the *Journal of the American Medical Women's Association* is devoted to this topic.

Chapter 6
FAMILY RESPONSIBILITIES
and career commitments

"I like to think that even though we're married, we're still
independent"
(Male physician)

When women physicians are compared with other highly educated
women, their patterns of marriage, divorce and motherhood are
similar – they marry later and less frequently than male physicians and
men in similar professions, they divorce more often, and they have
fewer children (Rosow and Rose 1972).[1] These statistics make it seem
as if high-status careers and marriage are intrinsically incompatible for
women in the United States. The usual reason given is the conflict
between two demanding roles. Another, less obvious, reason professional women marry later and not as often, and have a higher rate of
divorce and lower rate of remarriage than men of the same occupational status is our culture's prescription that women should "marry up."
Women are supposed to marry men who are better educated than they
are (as well as taller and older), but more important, men who have or
will have careers that are more prestigious and better paying. This
pattern is a holdover from the days when the husband was expected to
be the main breadwinner of the family. It also reflects the social
attitude that a man's ego will suffer badly if his wife outdistances him
occupationally.

For women physicians, as with other women in high-prestige
careers, there is no "up," except for novices marrying men further
along in their careers. Eventually the woman is likely to catch up, and
so, whether the status equality occurs in the early years, when medical

students marry, or in the later years, when the woman's training matches that of her husband, for most women in high-status professions, only marriage to a man of equally high occupational status is considered socially acceptable. Unfortunately, the pool of such eligible men is limited, and reduced even further because men of high status can marry women of lesser status, who thereby are marrying "up." This mandate of hypergamy that results in the lower rate of marriage among women of prestigious professional, educational, and social status, is called the "Brahmin effect," after the highest caste in India, whose women lose status if they marry lower-caste men.

The data on the marital status and number of children of the men and women in my two samples reflect these patterns. More men than women were married, and the men had more children (see *Tables 4 and 5*).

When comparing the lives of married male and female physicians, one must compare the traditional marriage, where the husband has a full-time career, and the wife is a housewife or does part-time or volunteer work, and the dual-career marriage, where both husband and wife have careers that demand high levels of professional commitment.[2] Since very few women physicians are married to househusbands or to men with minimal job demands, we are comparing men and women in dual-career marriages with men in traditional marriages.

The effects of marriage: "It's particularly nice to come home to one's spouse"

Traditionally married men see mostly beneficial effects from being married. As one young man who married during his internship said:

> During training when one works very, very hard and the free hours are very few, it's particularly nice to come home to one's spouse. When one gets depressed and tired, and the two seem to go hand in hand, it's very nice to have somebody who means a lot to you around. Somebody to share the time that you have.

In a similar circumstance, the effect of marriage on a woman physician in training can be quite different. One woman now in her fifties said:

> Before we were married, we had it worked out that I would have a three-year residency, at least, but it didn't turn out that way.

81

Table 4   *Family responsibilities of matched sample of respondents to AAMC 1976 longitudinal survey of class of 1960*

	males		females	
	no.	%	no.	%
marital status				
married	257	88.6	61	62.9
divorced or separated	22	7.6	14	14.4
widowed	3	1.0	4	4.1
never married	8	2.8	18	18.6
total	290	100.0	97	100.0
no. of children				
0	17	5.9	27	27.8
1	18	6.2	8	8.2
2	78	27.0	26	26.8
3+	176	60.9	36	37.1
total	289	100.0	97	99.9[1]
degree of family responsibility[2]				
low	19	6.5	25	25.8
medium	96	33.0	23	23.7
high	176	60.5	49	50.5
total	291	100.1	97	100.0

Notes: [1] Because of rounding, not all total percentages add up to 100.

[2] Female physicians were asked more specific questions in the Longitudinal Survey about the effect of family structure on career development than were male respondents. The family responsibility index for females consisted of the following variables: marital status, number of children, and responsibility for housework. The index of family responsibility for female physicians ranged from 0, indicating never married and no children, to 4, indicating married, with three or more children, and having primary responsibility for housework. Questions on responsibility for housework were not asked of male respondents; therefore the index of family responsibility for male physicians, which ranged from 0 to 3, represents their marital status and number of children. For the women, the scores were trichotomized as follows: Low (0–1), medium (2), high (3–4). For the men, low (0–1), medium (2), high (3).

He was very unhappy with the demands. Since we were married much over the objections of his parents, who felt that a career woman was not going to take good care of their boy, it got rough. He decided that he would go home and stay with his mother, and

Table 5   *Marital status and number of children of male and female physicians in interview study*

	males		females	
	no.	%	no.	%
marital status				
married	27	87	21	64
divorced	0	0	1	3
widowed	2	6	1	3
never married	2	6	10	30
total	31	99[1]	33	100
number of children[2]				
0	3	10	6	26
1	4	14	3	13
2	15	52	7	30
3+	7	24	7	30
total	29	100	23	99[1]

Notes: [1] Because of rounding, not all total percentages add up to 100.
[2] Married or formerly married only.

I could call him up when I was ready to come home and be a wife. That night the diaphragm came out, and my daughter was born nine months later. I was offered an assistant residency because the chief of medicine didn't know I was pregnant, but I didn't take it. Not having had the residency, I was not qualified to go on in any major capacity.

In contrast, a two-physician couple who married and had their children during medical school had a great deal of support, in all ways, from the wife's family of women physicians. As the husband, now in his forties, described it:

My wife's mother and grandmother were both physicians so they had a tradition of women physicians, and an interest in supporting us. My mother-in-law had a wing of the house which used to be her office, and we lived in that wing. There was not only the help of my in-laws, but people came as housekeepers, so we were very fortunate.

As long as they were in structured situations such as medical school, postgraduate training, and fellowships, they did not feel circumscribed by the children's needs and were able to relocate easily.

By the time their career demands proliferated, their children were already independent.

After training, the effects of marriage on the careers of the male physicians in traditional marriages continue to be advantageous, with the only restraint that of geographical mobility. Married male physicians get active support from their wives in many ways. One of the men interviewed had gone to medical school in his late twenties at his wife's urging. Another, who had been dissatisfied with general practice, was able to get a fellowship in chemotherapy and become a clinical researcher in oncology through a physician his wife had once worked for. Such support can be important throughout a physician's career. As one physician in his fifties said of his wife's approval of his career decisions:

> I have been fortunate in having a wife who was supportive of the requirements of the life of a medical researcher. It was far from regular, and not very well paid for a long time. I think that a wife probably makes the ultimate decision, whether you stay in the sort of work that you want to do but aren't necessarily producing a great deal in terms of finances.

While men's medical careers generally benefit from their being married, not all of their marriages benefit from those careers. Several male physicians I interviewed talked of their wives' estrangement, alcoholism, and even suicide.

Most women physicians in the United States who are not married to physicians are married to other professionals or to business executives. Being married to a man with a good income gives a woman physician freedom to be as active professionally as suits her. One woman I interviewed was in her forties and had limited her commitments. She said, "I have my household, my children, and my work. I don't have to be so busy, so I don't advertise myself." Another was in her thirties and trying to build up a private specialty practice. She was able to survive financially because her husband was a successful banker.

While a wife's earnings are important to her family's income (Oppenheimer 1977), to be the chief financial support of her husband is not considered socially legitimate. The long-accepted pattern of women working to put their husbands through medical school is seen as an investment in their own future as the wife of a successful professional. Once past the early career years, it is rare that the wife is the main breadwinner. For example, in one two-physician marriage, the wife felt her husband had not worked very hard because she was enough of a go-getter to support their family. The husband's emotional stability suffered, and the couple were eventually divorced. Another woman interviewed had juggled a demanding practice and the care of small children in the absence of her husband, but was unable to sustain the marriage when her husband came back from World War II to start over in private practice. In her words:

> I really think if it hadn't been for the war, my marriage wouldn't have broken up. It was a terrible rat race for me. I had two other doctors' practices that I was trying to hold for them – my husband's and our partner. I had two children who were at that point aged two and a few months and one and a few months. I had more than I could handle. When my husband came back, he was looking to me for a tremendous amount of support because he had had a rough time. I was looking to him for a lot of support because I had had a rough time. It was a three-ring circus – the patients, the children, my husband. I think my husband got the raw deal. I felt so guilty about it – like I had failed.

As for the overall effects of marriage on women physicians' careers, like men, they suffer from geographical restrictions, but unlike men, older women were inclined to sacrifice their careers to the demands of their marriages. One woman, now in her fifties, was married to a man who was a successful international lawyer despite an illness that left him disabled a few years after they married. She followed her husband around the world, took care of the children, maintained their households, and worked at salaried positions in nursing homes and employee health services. Yet even she said of her life:

> It worked out very, very well. I've kept my maiden name in the career. I enjoy the independence it's given me in my own thinking about myself. It has made absolutely no difference to how we behaved at home because we were married in the days when the man was the head of the house, and that's all there was to it, and that's the way it stayed. I don't think we are going to change now.

Another woman physician in her fifties, married to a physician, was bitter about her career sacrifices. She had been told by a male family friend before she entered medical school "that to fulfill yourself completely as a woman, you want to marry and have children, and you don't want to pull your husband around like a puppy on a string. You have to go where he goes." She married while she and her husband were still in medical school, a year apart. He was in the Navy when she graduated, and she gave up her choice of specialty and a highly prized internship to be with him. After World War II, they both did research at the same medical center, and had a nanny for their two children. After several years, her husband wanted to go into private practice in the small town where he was born, and where he had family property. She gave up her work to follow him, even though, she said:

> I never wanted to go. I thought it was the end of the world culturally, academically, intellectually. It was stultifying. Geographically, it was depressing. I just really didn't want to go.

The best medical clinic in town, which he had been invited to join, would not allow her to practice with them, nor would they keep him if she set up a competitive private practice. At that point, she said:

> I just really dug in my heels and said, "If you choose to go and absolutely deny my existence, go alone. I won't go under those circumstances." Well, there he sacrificed his career in that he didn't join the clinic, and we went into practice together. It was heavy to be working with him. The only time that he would have off, I would cover for him, if he had to go to a medical meeting, or to the naval reserve. It was really a bad segment. I would have to cover his rounds, his patients, my patients, the office, the family, the house, everything, and it was really too much.

They subsequently got a partner, and she then left the practice to work as a college physician and saw adolescent patients in a part-time private practice. She had two more children, and, in order to be accepted by the women of the community, she said:

> I worked fiendishly as a Girl Scout leader, as a Brownie leader, as a Camp Fire leader. I became head of the women's division of the opera company, and I was on the program committee for the PTA. I played bridge with the women in the afternoon, and I would surreptitiously be doing my practice in the morning.

After about ten years, they came back to the city and the medical center where they had originally worked. He went into clinical research and she became head of the employee health service, which she built up into a large unit with several physicians and a research program in occupational medicine.

Both these women illustrate the battle some women physicians fought to have some sort of career in the face of enormous marital demands during a period when women were supposed to put their careers last. Women under forty experience mutuality and reciprocity in career choices because their careers have legitimacy in the eyes of their husbands, families, colleagues, and in the larger society. Many younger women physicians are married to physicians, and their careers and family lives are subject to the particular advantages, constraints, and challenges of two-physician marriages.

Two-physician marriage:
"We don't have to translate into simple English"

In the United States, the increasing number of women going to medical school has produced a similarly increasing number of physicians married to physicians, to the extent that one writer commented, "If the trend continues with the new tidal wave of women physicians, it is not inconceivable that within a very few years the majority of young physicians either will be women doctors or will be married to one" (Fletcher 1982: 6).[3] The trend of physicians marrying physicians could have been predicted from two common social patterns – the pressure for women to marry men of at least equal status, and the likelihood of falling in love with the boy or girl "next door." Given the hermetically intense atmosphere of medical training, what would need explaining in these days of co-ed medicine is how physicians marry anyone *but* physicians!

The two-physician marriage has many similarities with any other dual-career marriage, such as the problem of choosing a geographical location that will give each spouse adequate career opportunities. The medical dual-career couple does have options of specialty choice and type of practice that afford a welcome measure of flexibility. The demands on dual-doctor couples are compounded by patients' needs, but medicine is not the only "greedy occupation" (Nadelson and Nadelson 1980; Handy 1978). In comparison, being able to have someone who understands one's work is one of the main advantages of being married to a physician.[4] The importance of being able to talk over problems at home was expressed by one male physician in a two-physician marriage this way:

> It's a real advantage to be in somewhat similar fields. It makes it easier for each of us to talk about what we're doing and for each of us to understand what problems, pressures, satisfactions, whatever, in the other's career are. We don't have to translate into simple English and use three times as many words to describe what is going on.

87

A male physician in his fifties, who had had both a traditional and a dual-career marriage, had this to say about the difference:

My first wife was a housewife. She was a quiet person and took care of my kids – our kids – and ran the house. I don't know what impact she had on my career except to be very patient with me when I came home late at night. My second wife works with me. She's a biochemist and runs the research laboratory. She has a lot of impact on my professional life because she is another dimension in my thinking. She knows the field well and we talk over a lot of problems. I think we help each other a great deal.

Meshing careers:
"I thought I was making a large sacrifice"

During the early years in two-physician marriages, the couples' main problem is to mesh their training locations. Among the twenty-seven physicians married to doctors that I interviewed, older women followed their husbands, but in the younger couples, the selection of location and timing of moves were mutual.

Non-physician wives are major influences in their husbands' career choices (Skipper and Gliebe 1977). In two-physician marriages, the husband and wife influence each other's choice of specialty and type of practice. In one couple, an older, already established obstetrician–gynecologist had urged his wife not to go into his specialty, which had been her first choice, but to go into internal medicine, which he felt was more prestigious. In another couple, the husband's concern was that his wife choose a specialty that would be compatible with having children and a family life. She had been offered a residency in dermatology, which was not a specialty she had considered, and her husband suggested she try it out. Her account reflects the subtleties of his influence:

My husband urged me not to do something like pediatrics. He is a very rational person. This was a thing that would be difficult for me if we wanted to have a family. He would have let me do what I wanted to do. It's not a dictatorial kind of thing, but he sort of reasoned with me, and said, "Why don't you try it?" And then I did become interested in it. It has worked out. I'm very, very happy now. I didn't have children then, and I didn't have them for a long time. Now I have four children. I had them all together. I couldn't be a surgeon or an obstetrician and still do a good job. I can do a good job as a dermatologist.

In a reversal of the usual pattern, the careers of the wives of the two of the younger men were further advanced than their husbands' when they married, and the men stayed in cities where their wives were already established. In one of these cases, the wife was a few years older than her husband, and she influenced him to change his plans about a fellowship and about his future specialty. His fellowship was to have been at Harvard, and his physician father was quite upset over his son's change of career plans. As it turned out, the young man's career took an upward turn because he went into an undermanned field, and was able to get a full-time staff position immediately. In his words:

> I had already lined up an excellent fellowship, and I decided to give that up. This was a major sacrifice that I made for her – for our relationship. It's been a very beneficial effect, in that I moved into a field where I was needed, unknowingly. I didn't really choose my specialty on that basis, but as it turned out, it was a very good decision, from a practical standpoint. A job was immediately available, and I was there to fill it, and it was a good job. It was very beneficial, but at the time I thought I was making a large sacrifice. I was changing my field for my wife and staying in this city for my wife.

In choosing whether they will go into an office practice or into academic medicine, in addition to considering their own proclivities and opportunities, physicians married to physicians usually strive for a balance of professional demands. If the husband is already in a busy entrepreneurial practice, the wife may choose a career in academic medicine. In one case, both the husband and the wife chose academic medicine because they had five children and wanted careers with controllable time demands. Balance in career type does not always solve the problems of conflicting priorities in a two-physician marriage. One woman in academic medicine married to a man with an office practice reported how she had to fight continuously for her professional needs. She said:

> We go away on weekends with the two small children. When we're attending physicians on a ward, we have a certain responsibility to that ward. We like to show up on weekends and make rounds with the residents. In our house, there's never

any question when my husband's attending on the ward that we stay in the city, so he can make rounds. And yet when it's my turn to make rounds, everyone is completely amazed and surprised that I want to stay here on Saturday and Sunday and make rounds. And it happens over and over again.

Collegiality and competition:
"It certainly has not unmade my career"

In compensation for the closing off of career options, both the husband and wife in a two-physician marriage gain a colleague who can be a powerful ally, since they become part of each other's referral and sponsorship networks (Lorber 1982). In one case, a wife was able to help her husband through a career change "with a few phone calls from *her* chief of service." In another instance, a husband who was involved in a political conflict was able to gain the support of the head of the department of internal medicine through his wife's well-placed position in the department. Another male physician, ironically, reaped the benefit of the women's movement through his wife. He said:

> Within the last three or four years, there has been a great interest in involving women and minorities in everything. Science and medicine have been no exception to this rule. So, consequently, my wife has been extremely active in a number of committees. Frequently, invitations have come to me through her committees when they're searching for some resource. They will have learned through my wife of my talents, or, in fact, if she's been invited to lecture in a city, frequently as part of just being a good host, the person who's invited her will say, "What is your husband interested in?" Then I will get a call from someone in my field who'll say, "I understand you're coming out, and we would like to have you talk or see patients, and do whatever." This accounts for about 10 or 15 or 20 per cent of my contacts. I find it hard to tell you if it made my career, but I can tell you it certainly has not unmade my career.

In addition to these examples of explicit help, there were instances of implicit aid. In one case, a young physician, whose wife was already established when they married, seemed to have been the beneficiary of the hospital's desire to retain her on their staff. Without anything said openly, and without his asking, he was given a full-time staff appointment and patient privileges immediately after his fellowship was completed. He was surprised by the ease with which he was appointed, since he had done all of his earlier training elsewhere. He said:

> My wife's career, at the point when we got married, was advancing. The man with whom I was working indicated that he would be happy to have me stay here. He didn't really say so – he just kept appointing me, and every year, I would get an appointment for the following year.

This "gentleman's agreement" had a negative side. His wife commented in her interview that when job offers come for the two of them, "It's kind of amusing, because usually there is some fantastic job for one person, and the other person's offer is either marginal or trumped up." Thus, while hidden aid may be palatable at the beginning, it may not stay hidden as careers develop and may become unacceptable to couples of markedly different professional attainments, especially when the wife is the more successful one.

However, competition does not seem to be an overt problem, even with husbands and wives in parallel careers. I interviewed a couple who were both in academic medicine, at the same stages of their careers, and working in different units in the same building. They had been married when they were both in their thirties and finished with their training. At the time of their interviews, they were both directing research and publishing frequently, and both expressed similar high aspirations for their professional futures. Since it is the men in dual-career marriages who have been reported to be most concerned with competition and relative status (Holmstrom 1972; S.M. Miller 1971; Poloma and Garland 1971), I asked the husband whether he felt competitive with his wife, and if he did, what effect this had on his career. He said:

> I consider my wife certainly my equal, if not my superior; I have the same competitive feelings about her that I do to anyone else at that level. The effects are only positive. Having been married has been very good to me, not only socially and personally, but professionally, in that my competitive nature is now on all day and all night long, and I'm like a finely tuned athlete. I always consider it a privilege being married to her. I think that's been one spinoff I never recognized. It's been just delightful. I feel this competitiveness has really been a warm, nice feeling. It's made it easier for me to be competitive in other situations. I

don't have any anger or regrets in this competitiveness and I consider it only natural.

One constraint on dual-doctor marriages is the difficulty of working in the same institution as a spouse and keeping professional identities separate. This was the problem of a couple recently appointed to the same institution. They were doing research and seeing patients in different units, and used different names. Yet, the husband complained, even the mail clerks knew they were married as soon as they arrived, and in everything, from their mail to their demands for more office space, they were lumped together. He said:

Both of us, since we've arrived here, are developing further, requiring more space. We're almost simultaneously demanding more space and support. Now the attitudes of some of the people that we have to interact with, is that they cannot separate us in their minds, even though we are independent individuals who happen to be married, but pursuing independent careers. I will go and speak to an individual, and I'll be talking to him about my demands, and on occasion, my wife's demands filter into the conversation – not brought up by me, but brought up by this other individual whose attitude is based on a more rigid way of looking at married people. I find that difficult to deal with. We're professionally not a team. We're professionally independent. I like to think that even though we're married, we're still independent.

But this physician also said one of the advantages of being married to a physician was the intangible effect of being able to discuss the politics involved in academic medicine. He said, "She's very helpful in my strategy, in my writing, and doing my research, and dealing with some of the politics. I hope I contribute to her strategy as well." When couples work in the same institution, being treated as a team may be closer to reality than their insistence that they are quite separate and independent (Lorber 1979).

For both husband and wife, a marriage that creates an additional strand in the web of professional contacts is a decided advantage.[5] In general, the extent of "coupleness" depends on whether the husband and the wife are in the same colleague networks. As one wife said:

What happens is that the professional and the social get somewhat mixed together. Most of our social contacts have some professional contacts as well. We even have some amusing sets of friends where one of us is friendly with the husband and the other with the wife because of a professional contact. In one case, I'm friendly with the husband, and my husband is friendly with the wife. I collaborate with the man and he collaborates with the woman.

Such combined professional socializing also eases the time pressures on a dual-career couple, but it may be at the price of professional independence.

The effects of children:
"An enormous asset to life"

There is no doubt that the addition of children to a couple creates an entirely new constellation of relationships and coping patterns. For male physicians in traditional marriages, children are an enrichment to their lives and make few demands other than financial (Heins 1979). However, even in a dual-career marriage, a large family is manageable. One couple in their thirties married before they entered medical school. Their first child was born in their second year, the next in their fourth year. The third child was born when he was working in a research institute, and she was head of a county health department. The fourth was born during the wife's fellowship, and the fifth when both were attending physicians in hospital-based practices. Both had deliberately chosen specialties and types of careers that were not time-pressured in order to be able to spend time with the children. In his words:

It's actually been pretty easy because we've always been in the same institution. We've never had any real conflicts in terms of time. There have really been no problems. I'm an only child, and I have to admit that with the birth of each one, I had heart failure and thought we would never make it through. My wife wanted six children or more, and it's worked out remarkably well. Financially, it's been a strain now and then, and it may eventually influence what I do. I may branch out into private practice just to increase my income. It would be a little disappointing to have to give up research.

As this physician indicated, for male physicians, the problem children present tends to be mostly financial. For women physicians, the problem is the allocation of time. If there are compromises to be made in spending time at work or with their children, they, rather than their husbands, make them. One woman in her thirties in an academic career, married to a physician in private practice, said:

> If I weren't married and didn't have children, I think I would have a different type of career. At the moment, my life is fairly structured so that I can work from 9 to 6 with minimal work on weekends and night duty. I think if I didn't have children and didn't have a husband, I would probably be working the evenings and working the weekends. I'd be in private practice, and one reason I am not doing that kind of work is because I am married and have children, that's for sure.

A woman in her forties with four children was in private practice, but in a specialty with controllable time demands. She said:

> No matter what you say, you compromise somewhat along the line. I've compromised in my choice of specialty, and I compromise in the time I spend in my practice. I made some sacrifices, and I know how important it is for you to have a compromise.

When asked if her husband, a child psychiatrist, made similar compromises for the children, she said, "I would say not too much, no. He helps out a bit, but compromise his career, I would say not."

Another woman in her forties, an extremely successful researcher with two children, also married to a physician, had given up leisure-time activities in order to devote time to both work and her children. In her words:

> There is no doubt that if you have children and do anything that's appropriate as far as rearing them, it takes a chunk of effort, but whether it is a chunk that would have been spent in effective work, I think is questionable. It's a matter of whether or not you're willing to give up a certain amount of *free* time that you might have had at one point, time to read, or do whatever you like to do, and devote *that* time to your children. Or whether you insist on continuing to have that kind of time and the children and do your professional work, too. I think that if you do the latter, you detract from your work effort. If you do the former, it means you give up your free time and call your children your hobby. I consider children an enormous asset to life. I think they are an absolute joy, and I like to spend time with them.

Family responsibilities and career commitments

The question of how children fit into a dual-career marriage depends on whether they are considered work or pleasure, and whose responsibility their child-care and financial needs fall to. The general pattern among couples in their thirties and forties is that the overall financial responsibility is the husband's and the overall child-care responsibility the wife's. If a sacrifice has to be made for financial reasons, such as giving up an academic career to go into a more lucrative private practice, that sacrifice will be the husband's. If a sacrifice of work or leisure time has to be made to be the emotionally sustaining parent to the children, that sacrifice will be the wife's.

The work-family role system

According to Joseph Pleck, the work-family role system is composed of the male work role, the female work role, the female family role, and the male family role (Pleck 1977, 1983). In a traditional marriage, the male work role involves not only the time spent in actual work, but also professional socializing after work, attending committee meetings, out-of-town travel, keeping up with recent developments, and so on. The female family role similarly involves not only actual home maintenance and child care, but attendance at school meetings, taking the children to doctors and dentists, running the children's and the couple's social lives, sustaining kinship and religious obligations, participating in community voluntary activities, and so on. The female work role is secondary to her family role in time and involvement, and the male family role is to "help" and spend leisure time with the children. The wife's income is secondary to the economic wherewithal of the family, but the husband's career advancement enhances his family's financial and social status.

This division of labor by gender in the "two-person single career" (Papanek 1973) is so pervasive in our society that the ideal solution for dual-career couples has frequently been to find a housekeeper "wife" so that both the man and the woman can pursue the male type of work role. The more common compromise is a patchwork of servants, baby-sitters, schools, and after-school activities that do not offer the freedom from home-care responsibility that a traditional wife (or "jewel" of a housekeeper) gives. The wife's income is likely to pay for childcare and housekeeping arrangements, and she is usually the one to organize these substitutes for what is seen as her responsibility. Even in seemingly egalitarian dual-career marriages, the wife has the worrying responsibility of home maintenance and child care. As a sociologist married to a physician said of his "lapsed egalitarianism":

> I guess what dismays me and makes me see my marriage and family as unfortunately typically upper-middle-class collegial, pseudo-egalitarian American – especially in light of my own continuing commitment to an egalitarian, participatory ethos – is that I assume no responsibility for major household tasks and family activities. True, my wife has always worked at her profession (she is a physician), even when our sons were some weeks old. (I used to say that behind the working wife with young children, there stands a tired husband.) True, I help in many ways and feel responsible for her having time to work at her professional interests. But I do partial, limited things to free her to do her work. I don't do the basic thinking about the planning of meals and housekeeping, or the situation of the children. Sure, I will wash dishes and "spend time" with the children; I will often do the shopping, cook, make beds, "share" the burden of most household tasks; but that is not the same thing as direct and primary responsibility for planning and managing a household and meeting the day-to-day needs of children.
>
> (S.M. Miller 1971: 37)

In short, beneath the egalitarian overlay of the coping patterns of many dual-career couples with children is a traditional division of responsibility.[6]

In contrast to solutions that depend solely on the couple's own individual resources, one woman physician took advantage of the communal services her hospital gave to medical students and housestaff to create an innovative solution to home maintenance. Now in her fifties, she had married a non-physician during medical school, with the agreement that she would not cook or do housework. During her postgraduate training, she arranged her home life so that it revolved around the hospital. As she described it:

> We had an apartment across the street, and it made life easy. We ate in the cafeteria, and then later when the children came, I could be home for lunch, and while the nursemaid was taking care of them, see them during the few hours in-between my duties. The pediatrician was in the same apartment building. It was, all in all, the best kind of arrangement.

She later had an office nearby and an affiliation in the same hospital, so she continued "the proximity of all the activities." Thus, by taking advantage of the dormitory housing and common meals offered to all students, this married women physician was able to provide her family with a support system that did not totally depend on her and her husband.

Many medical centers and universities in the United States have long provided living quarters, cafeterias, laundry and cleaning services for students and house staff. Employee health services are also usually available in large work organizations. Child-care centers are rarer, but can be found in some workplaces. It would not be a radical step to make all these services widely available, in the style of the Israeli kibbutz or the Chinese commune, at workplaces and schools throughout the United States. As described by Ruth Sidel in *Women and Child Care in China*, the model would be something like the Institute for Biological Products in Peking. It is, she says:

[a] self-contained neighborhood including laboratories for scientific work, dormitories for single workers, quarters for married workers, dining halls, a nursery and a primary school,…and many kinds of people living together who are needed to service the institute – gardeners, grandparents, teachers, medical personnel, scientists, and mechanics. It is a true neighborhood, with large trees, paths leading from the work area to the living quarters and to the nursery, all within easy walking distance. A married worker with children can go to the dining hall for breakfast, drop her child at the nursery, walk to work, return to the dining hall for lunch, work the rest of the day, pick up the child at the nursery, and then either eat with her family in the dining hall or make dinner for them at home.[7]

(Sidel 1972: 32)

Private solutions to dual work and family role responsibilities that augment the wife with hired help do not challenge the traditional sexual division of labor. Few wives in dual-career marriages are as free of family responsibilities as their husbands are. They are adept at working full-time, with high professional commitment, and running their households, too (Heins *et al.* 1976). But what they find extremely difficult to fit in, especially when their children are small, is the "third job" – the professional socializing and informal contacts that are so crucial to career advancement. If men, both in traditional and in seemingly egalitarian dual-career marriages are freer to spend their time cultivating contacts and colleagues, then the pattern of women not advancing to the highest levels of their professions will be perpetuated.

Notes

1 According to unpublished US Bureau of Labor Statistics Current Population Survey data for March, 1983, based on 60,000 households, 82.7 per cent of the men and 63.6 per cent of the women in health-diagnosing occupations are married and living with their spouses; 10.9 per cent of the men and 26.3 per cent of the women have never been married; and 3.9 per cent of the men and 11 per cent of the women are divorced.

2 For studies of dual-career marriages see Fava and Genovese 1983; Yogev 1982; Hunt and Hunt 1982, 1977; Pepitone-Rockwell 1980; Hall and Hall 1979; Bryson and Bryson 1978; Berman, Sacks, and Lief 1977; Rapoport and Rapoport 1976; and Rice 1979.

3 Two-physician marriages are so popular in the United States that Drs Esther and David Nash formed a national organization, Dual Doctor Families, to represent their interests. The organization publishes a newsletter, compiles bibliographies, and sponsors research (see Staver 1983).

4 For glowing accounts of marriage to women physicians by their husbands, see Eisenberg 1981; Nadelson and Eisenberg 1977; Aronson 1974.

5 Epstein found the same pattern among women lawyers (1981: 340–43). For a woman, marriage to another professional, whether in the same occupation or not, makes it more likely that she will be included in the social activities of her male colleagues (Kaufman 1978).

6 Similar observations are made by Pleck 1983; Angell 1982, 1981; Poloma and Garland 1971.

7 Of course, one hopes that if Utopia comes, this married worker will as often be a "he" as a "she."

Chapter 7
RETROSPECTS AND PROSPECTS:
the crossroads turn

"Life has pretty well dictated what I did"
(Woman physician)

Successful careers in medicine are built on a combination of sponsorship, visibility, and reciprocal favors. These factors build on each other, and as careers develop, they frequently have crucial points at which a physician is set on the road to higher professional status or a downward spiral starts.[1] These "crossroads turns," as one female physician termed them, may or may not be recognized while they are happening. Frequently, only when looking back is it evident when the opportune moment was seized or missed. Sometimes an outside observer can better see the locus and timing of significant career determinants. The overall perspective of this book shows that motivation and ambition can goad a physician to seek out a situation which will make the best use of his or her potential, but also demonstrates that personal qualities, while necessary, are not sufficient for success.

Career trajectories are shaped by personal decisions within a structure of opportunities and a climate of social attitudes. The social climate influences what possibilities are envisaged, and these in turn influence personal decisions. Demands of training institutions, workplaces, the job market, and families further limit options. Type of medical school and prestige of postgraduate education are powerful sorting and tracking mechanisms for novice physicians in the United States. After training, the setting within which a physician works supplies varying resources, stimulation, contacts, and helps and hindrances from colleagues and gatekeepers (For similar processes in other types of work, see Lin, Ensel, and Vaughn 1981; Lin, Vaughn, and Ensel 1981; Granovetter 1974).

The older generation:
the need for challenge

Male physicians in their forties and fifties who are the most successful have been able to take advantage of their location in places where stimulating research was being done, and where there was a proliferation of both money for research and referrals of private patients. Men who had to overcome enmity among superiors and detrimental organizational reshuffling are less successful but most survive professionally. The least successful are those who found themselves in backwater units, and who did not have the personal qualities to get out or change their situations.

The importance of the work situation for a man of middling capabilities is illustrated by a cardiologist who was able to learn his specialty and do research and administrative work when he was appointed to run the cardiology service in a municipal hospital affiliated with the voluntary hospital where he had privileges. When the voluntary hospital pulled out of the arrangement, he returned to full-time practice and felt his career took a downward turn. He said:

When I ran that division, my learning ability took a huge spurt. Then, when that stopped, my learning abilities have kind of tapered down. I think that if physicians who are in practice would continue to be challenged, they would to a better job.

For the older generation of women physicians, the work situation is even more of a make-or-break factor. This cohort of women physicians particularly needed colleague support to be productive and recognized for their work. Without it, they fade professionally. If they are in stimulating settings with excellent professional resources, they are successful; if they are not, they flounder. As one woman in her fifties, who was in a low-keyed and marginal unit in a research oriented hospital, said:

I have twenty-two unwritten papers in which all the work is done and analyzed, but I've never written them. It just happened that everyone I've ever been with has allowed me to do that. They never cared whether I wrote a paper or not. Everywhere I've been they've always given me a lot of support to do anything I wanted to do, allowed me to do it, been interested in the results as they come out, but nobody has ever said to me that you've got to write that up. I've never once in my career been told that. I just never had the self-discipline to do it. I somehow think that had I been made to do it earlier, if it had been demanded of me earlier in my development, it might have come easier.

Another woman also recognized that not leaving a position where she was stagnating stymied her professional development:

I should have gone somewhere else after two or three years on the staff. I should have gone into an active research group where it would have been much easier to do research. I could have just looked for another job. I didn't and I think that was a mistake. I've been here for all of my professional career, and I probably should have gone somewhere else.

A woman who did leave an unrewarding work situation felt she had turned around her career. She left an office-based practice that gave her too little professionally and economically for the long days she was putting in. She took a job as assistant director of an employee health service in a large organization where she saw a variety of medical problems and had the respect of her colleagues. She described the difference in these two work situations as follows:

I had gone to fine pre-med and medical schools, I was a well-trained doctor, and it seemed to me I was physically killing myself with not nearly the economic reward that I thought I should be getting. Here, it's very satisfying. It's intellectually and academically stimulating. It's like a little town – I feel like a small-town personal physician.

She was extremely happy with the decision. It was, she felt, a major turning point in her career and gave her satisfying rewards for her capabilities.

Another case illustrates how the same person can flourish or be held back, depending on the work situation. One woman with a productive career in academic medicine had been appointed to her first full-time staff position by the outgoing chief of service before he was replaced by a sexist chief. She said:

I got appointed as an attending just at the time the old chief was leaving. He used to like me because we would chat over coffee. The new chief distinctly did not want females. He never outright said it, but it took me four years until he accepted me as equally worthy as my male counterparts.

Not until she was accepted was she able to bloom professionally.

The younger generation:
"Time for paying in dues"

The training period sets many male physicians well on their way professionally, whereas women must often fight for career advantages in their first work situations. A male physician with a good staff appointment in a research-oriented setting had started a project in college and continued it in medical school, and it helped get him his current position in a research unit. As he said, "Things I've done in the past have led to one decision at a time that has led here." Another young male physician had had a fellowship in what he called a "fair-haired department," and was able to stay on to continue his research. As he said, "It's been a nice ride so far." Like older male physicians who built their careers through sponsorship which recognized their competence, these physicians had gone from residencies to fellowships to staff appointments with the help of contacts they made along the way. The contacts gave them referrals and consultations if they were in office practice, and money for research and laboratory resources if they were in academic medicine.

Even men who do not have prestigious early training are able to rapidly overcome their initial handicap. A US citizen who graduated from a foreign medical school and did an internship in Canada found a fellowship in hematology and oncology in a hospital in the United States through an advertisement in a medical journal. There, he worked with someone who knew the chief of medicine in his current location. This connection got him his current position, where he was running a laboratory, doing research, writing, lecturing, and building a small private practice. Another male physician who had a circuitous route to a good position had not gotten into medical school the first time he applied. He had planned to go into office practice, but he chose a stint at the National Institutes of Health in lieu of military service. That gave him a chance to do research, and he met people who sponsored him for his current position on the staff of a prestigious research-oriented hospital.

In contrast, women with good training still have to struggle for a professional foothold. One physician interviewed was working extremely hard to prove to her colleagues that having a newborn baby was not going to cut into her professional commitments. Another was in a burgeoning sub-specialty in a unit where she was the only physician, so she was in a good position to administer and build up the department. Her plans were to do so, as well as to teach, do research, and consult, but she will have to reach outside of her immediate work situation for colleague support. A third young woman in academic medicine, whose first staff appointment was obtained with the help of the head of her research institute when she was a fellow, felt her position was shaky and that the best thing she could do at this point in her professional life was to accrue professional credits against her future. She said:

> A lot of what I'm doing right now is putting in a tremendous amount of work, partly with the thought that the more I produce now, the more options I have in a shorter period of time as to where I can go, and how good a place I go. I figure it's time for paying in my dues now.

Four women in their thirties were at crossroad turns at the time of the interview, and the prognosis was not good. One who was not doing well felt she had been too feminine and flirtatious in medical school and so had not been recommended for good post graduate training (Bourne 1977). She now wanted a hospital affiliation where she had not trained, which is an extremely unlikely prospect. She had aspirations for a more prestigious specialty practice than she was likely to have. She expressed her ambitions as follows:

> I want to gain the respect of my colleagues. I'd like to have doctors referring me their patients and their family, and I'll know from the kinds of referrals I'll be getting whether I'm succeeding.

Unfortunately, with her poor history during training, her reluctance to use the connections she already has, and her choice of a male-dominated specialty, it is doubtful that her aspirations will materialize.

Another young woman whose career was going downhill was a well-trained endocrinologist who did not get a full-time staff appointment in a research-oriented hospital. She had wanted a career in academic medicine, but she was being pushed into an entrepreneurial practice. In order to build up a clientele, she was dividing her time between her current affiliation and a more clinically oriented hospital where she had done a residency. She was unhappy about all the hustling she would have to do to make it in an office-based practice. Her ambivalence was expressed as follows:

I really didn't want to go into private practice and before you know it, there it was. But it's been surprisingly fun in a way I didn't expect it to be, and I would like to get more involved with patient care because I love to take care of patients, I really do. I just hadn't quite thought I would like the rigmarole of the paper work and the finances. I mean it's a big business, but I can't imagine that my practice would ever be a big business.

Two women in academic medicine were going nowhere because they were in work situations that gave them little encouragement, support, or stimulation. One had a weak and ineffective chief and was finding it difficult to write her own grant proposals, build up her referrals, or get salary increases or promotions. She had had a protected career, in which, she said, "I never had to fight." Now that she was faced with doing so, she was talking of leaving medicine entirely. Another woman who had been successful so far was in a peripheral department with a chief whose career had stagnated for many years. She knew she would have to leave in a year or two, but had not formulated where she wanted to go with any degree of clarity.

Future plans:
"I wish to stay like this for the next hundred years"

Most of the men interviewed were totally satisfied with their current situations, like the male physician who had changed his specialty and type of practice in his forties, and wanted now to do what he was doing "for the next hundred years." The younger men planned changes that would add to what they had already accomplished – a referral practice while continuing to do research in one case, technology development in addition to a thriving practice in another.

Younger women planned changes that might finally consolidate their careers. A dermatologist in her thirties planned to learn plastic surgery in the hope of expanding her practice; a cardiologist in the same age bracket planned to write a book for patients in the hope of getting more referrals. Two women physicians with unstable hospital staff appointments were thinking of what to do next: one was in the throes of a decision as to whether she would go into private practice, while the other thought she would like to work in an intensive care setting or in a non-specialized hospital.

Doing it over:
"The only thing I could have changed"

In looking back over their careers, men tend to have few regrets because they believe they have mostly been in charge of their careers. They feel their choices were good ones; if they were not, they learned from their mistakes, and were able to shift to better work situations. As one physician in his forties said:

> As far as training went, I don't think I would have done anything differently. I trained in very, very good institutions. I would have chosen nothing different. I picked up a specialty that has become very satisfying. I don't think I would have done things any differently. I'm happy with the way things are.

Women who are satisfied with their careers are relieved that things have turned out well. As one woman in her thirties said:

> It's funny because I always landed somewhere where I didn't want to be at the time, but it always worked out very well, and I enjoyed it. I don't think there's anything I would really change.

The only man who expressed a sentiment like that was one who had bowed to his wife's wishes and changed his specialty so they could live where she was already established as a physician. Also in his thirties, he said:

> I don't think it could have worked out any better. I don't think I would have gotten a better position than I have now. I was in the right place at the right time for this position.

He, like so many of the women, knew he had made his choices with limited options, and so was pleased that everything worked out well after all (Lovelace 1985). As one woman internist in her fifties, who had wanted to be a surgeon, said:

> When I was doing these things, that was the only way to do them. The professional scene was such that one couldn't have done it any other way. One could have a pipe dream but what would I have come out with thirty years later? I'm pretty happy with the way things have gone with my interests.

Women who knew when the detrimental turning points in their careers occurred often have major regrets about their past decisions. They realized early that the die was cast, and that they were locked into unrewarding careers. A woman physician who gave up a prestigious internship to follow her husband said, "I wouldn't have given away my power." But many felt that they had no choice but to do what they had done. Like some foreign-trained physicians, both women and men, who have to practice in specialties they feel are uncongenial when they come to the United States, women with deep regrets feel that the costs of fighting exclusion, blocked mobility, and family pressures were too great. In order to have any medical career at all, they had to practice in specialties and in settings where they were accepted (Fox and Richards 1977; Goldblatt and Goldblatt 1976).

Two of the women interviewed, both in their fifties, expressed the same sense of helplessness in the face of forces beyond their control. One, who had sacrificed her professional aspirations for her marriage, summed up the "cultural mandate" (Bourne and Wikler 1978). She said:

> I was not abnormal in 1940. It was abnormal for me to go on to medical school. It wasn't abnormal for me to accede to ordinary husbandly expectations. They weren't demands – they were just expectations. Life has pretty well dictated what I did.

The other woman was educated in a country where women physicians were not abnormal, but left for political reasons, only to face double discrimination in this country. She said:

> I would have probably enrolled in an American medical school and been an American graduate instead of a foreign graduate and gotten one obstacle away from my career. If you have three uncontrollable parameters in your life – being a woman, having an accent and a foreign diploma – that would have been the only thing I could have changed.

Main professional accomplishments:
"I've been able to get everything together"

In assessing what they accomplished during their careers, women tend to stress their value to patients, using words like "help" and "care." One woman in her fifties said, "I think the best thing I do is simply taking care of patients and being a warm and caring physician." Men tend to talk of their skills and their choice of appropriate treatment. A male physician in his fifties, assessing his accomplishments, said, "I became quite skillful in non-invasive cardiology and its applications." The personal side of the patient-physician relationship, being appreciated, even loved, is rarely mentioned by men.

In other areas of professional life, such as research, program development, career progress, teaching, and publications, male and female physicians describe their accomplishments in similar terms. Two physicians in their thirties with parallel accomplishments in academic medicine practices summed up their career progress in the same way. The male physician said he was proud of the following:

> Learning how to design treatment programs in patients with leukemia, learning how to take care of these diseases, being very confident when I have patients with these diseases and knowing how to take care of them. Writing some papers, being director of the laboratory. That's very satisfying to me. Being recognized in my small medical community as somebody who knows a lot about a certain area that he can help you with.

The woman physician said she took pride in these accomplishments:

> I can take care of a difficult hematology referral. I got all my boards done. And now four years out, I have enough experience so I am comfortable dealing with a referred hematology patient. I have some papers that I've written on the laboratory work side of things. I do a fair amount of teaching and run a couple of teaching programs.

Unrealistic aims lead to self-denigration of accomplishments. One woman in her forties with a career in clinical research felt she had not done anything she could be terribly proud of:

> Some great discovery that would get me the Nobel prize – anything else is not an accomplishment. I have people who say just taking care of patients and making them better is an accomplishment, but that's not out of the ordinary.

More realistic goals gave a dermatologist in her thirties a strong sense of pride when she attained them. She said:

> I've been able to get everything together. I consider I made it last year. I'm proud I made it by age thirty-three or thirty-four – being responsible and getting a big practice and handling it. I'm professionally well-liked by the community. I've gotten a big kick out of being put in *Who's Who in the East*.

There is a subtle interplay between self-expectations, accomplishments, and the recognition of others. Unrealistic goals are unlikely to be encouraged, but in the face of lack of encouragement, goals can be set too low. When others expect success, failures are often ignored as temporary lapses, but when others downgrade potential or ambitions, many successes are needed to establish the reputation of a high achiever. Those favored by the expectation of great accomplishment are likely to accomplish much; those hindered by the expectation of lesser accomplishment are likely to accomplish less. Of course there are always early "water walkers" who later drown, and "late bloomers" who produce astonishing fruit, but in the general pattern, the self-fulfilling prophecy is more influential in shaping professional careers that the ideology of equality of opportunity.

The informal organization of medicine and "Saturn's Rings"

The inequities in the informal organization of medicine that have blocked the advancement of women contradicts the belief that success is a matter of individual motivation and ambition and personal qualities. The career trajectories of the physicians interviewed show that professional development is as dependent on the actions of colleagues and superiors as on the person concerned. Too often, colleagues assume that if a person has not attained a high professional status, he or she did not want it, yet ambitions get thwarted and the offering of an opportunity creates possibilities that might otherwise be unimagined. As Oswald Hall said in 1946 in describing the process of sponsorship:

> Much of the assistance given by the sponsor to his protégé is of an intangible sort. It may be as nebulous as the help of an older person who encourages a younger person to define himself as a potential colleague. Since the professional ambition is, in its early stages, a fragile affair this aid is very important. However, the aid may be much more substantial. It may mean smoothing the path to easy acceptance to the right training school; it may mean appointments to positions within the appropriate institutions; it may mean deflecting clientele from the sponsor to the protégé; it may mean designating the protégé as successor to the sponsor.
>
> (Hall 1946: 152)

The aid of established physicians has been crucial to the career development of male physicians; it is no less, and indeed, probably more crucial to the career development of women physicians. For both men and women, sponsors help smooth the path in all the myriad ways novices become established members of their work worlds, but women in male-dominated occupations need the sponsorship of the established members of inner circles to document their worthiness as colleagues in the face of long-standing prejudices to the contrary. When they do not have strong sponsorship, their careers may stagnate, and very often, they do not know why. They tend to blame themselves, feeling they should have done things differently. They cannot put their finger on the source of their uneasiness with their career development, so they do not know exactly what they could have changed. As one woman in her thirties said:

> There are an awful lot of stupid little things that I would have done differently, but basically, the way everything turned out, there's nothing really major I would change. It would have to be a whole bunch of little tiny things that might have led to something different. No one big thing.

It is my suspicion that she is responding to the minutiae of sexism, what Mary Rowe called the "Saturn's rings phenomenon":

> These minutiae are usually not (practically speaking) actionable; most are such petty incidents that they may not even be identified, much less protested. They are, however, important, like the dust and ice in Saturn's rings, because, taken together, they constitute formidable barriers. As Saturn is partially obscured by its rings, so are good jobs practically obscured for minorities and women, by "grains of sand": the minutiae of discrimination.
> (Rowe 1977b: 56)[3]

The concept of Saturn's rings is doubly symbolic. Recent research in astronomy has shown that within the rings, particles are tracked into constant trajectories by gravity. In the work world, the need for trust and loyalty among colleagues, the grooming of protégés by sponsors, the differential evaluation of the potentials and achievements of women and men by gatekeepers, the accumulation of advantages and disadvantages in response to the halo of the Matthew effect or to Salieri-like denigration – all these pervasive practices lead to consistent career trajectories. The favored cluster in powerful inner circles, the acceptable hover around them in friendly colleague circles, and the rest drift in the outmost ring.

Notes

1 Daniel Levinson places the turning point for men at age forty. He says, "A man around forty has the experience of arriving at a culmination, a turning point. A specific event often serves as a marker indicating where he now stands and how far he can go. This *culminating event* represents some form of success or failure, of movement forward or backward on the life path" (Levinson 1978:31, author's emphasis). An earlier version of the same concept is:

> "There is a tide in the affairs of men,
> Which, taken at the flood, leads on to fortune;
> Omitted, all the voyage of their life
> Is bound in shallows and in miseries."

(Shakespeare, *Julius Ceasar* Act 4, Sc. 3,1. 218–21)

2 For similar processes in other types of work, see Lin, Ensel, and Vaughn 1981; Lin, Vaughn, and Ensel 1981; Granovetter 1974.

3 See also Bourne 1979.

Coda
STRATEGIES FOR CHANGE:
the paradox of feminist politics

"We'll see where the power goes"
(Woman physician)

It is extremely difficult to fight informal discrimination as an individual. Petty incidents and covert slurs can rarely be confronted outright. The most well-meaning people use long-standing assumptions about the proper roles and expected behavior of women and men without recognizing their discriminatory effect. The ideology of equal opportunity, fairness, and merit is accepted at face value, and it is an article of faith that competent and qualified women will make it as long as they are not formally excluded. When they don't, the blame is placed on their personal choices.

Stars, such as Margaret Thatcher, Golda Meier, and Indira Ghandi, seemingly demonstrate the openness of opportunities to talented, hard-working women. Closer examination of their careers shows that they became trusted colleagues in male-dominated inner circles and were groomed for leadership by powerful male sponsors. Stars may become role models for other women, and may make it less difficult for men to accept women in positions of leadership, but they rarely challenge male domination directly by advancing other women as protégées or by fighting for changes in social institutions.

Supposedly, all that is needed to eradicate systematic gender inequality is to find and train more competent, qualified women. As they move through their careers, they will redress current imbalances, and in proportion to their numbers, the best of them will rise to the top. Although Rosabeth Moss Kanter predicted a qualitative change

111

in attitudes towards women as their numbers in a workplace increase (Kanter 1977b). Women are underrepresented in positions of leadership even where they are a majority of the workers (Poll 1978; Grimm and Stern 1974). Increasing the number of women in a male-dominated workplace can bring a backlash. As the number of women increases, they have less contact with male colleagues and less support from female supervisors (South *et al.* 1982b). Women's confidence in their abilities to succeed and to lead expands with a rise in their numbers (Izraeli 1983; Spangler, Gordon, and Pipkin 1978), but men become resistent to their competition and to the loss of dominant status (Goode 1982: 137).

The recognition that numbers alone are not the answer to gender inequality was well expressed by the comment of a woman physician in her forties who said, "I'm encouraged by all the young women who are going into medicine, but we'll see where the power goes." If women are to gain positions of power, the patterns of the informal organization of the workplace must *routinely* include them. As a group, women must be trusted as colleagues, sponsored for advancement, given recognition for competence and accomplishment, and accrue the resources and reciprocal favors that advance careers. Paradoxically, women must act politically as a group in order to defuse gender as a status.

The question has to be raised as to the ultimate goal of advancing women as a group. Is it simply to put more women into positions of power in existing institutions, or is it to change the structure of institutions and their values and practices to reflect women's special perspective? Do women have a different view of the world than men? To what extent can we speak of women as a monolithic group?

At the end of the nineteenth century, Elizabeth Blackwell and Mary Putnam Jacobi promulgated contrasting approaches for advancing the cause of women physicians. Blackwell, according to Regina Morantz, felt that women physicians should have "special responsibilities in order to achieve what she believed was a higher social and moral purpose. Women physicians were to be 'in' the profession but not 'of' it" (Morantz 1982a: 473; see also Hayes 1981). Jacobi, in contrast, "saw women participating in the profession, not as a distinct entity unto themselves, but as separate individuals united with men by objective, demonstrable, and professional criteria in the search for truth (Morantz 1982a: 473). In current feminist terms, Blackwell was a cultural feminist and a separatist, and Jacobi was a liberal feminist and an integrationist (Lorber 1981b).

In the nineteenth century, Dr Blackwell and other women physicians organized clinics and hospitals to serve what they saw as the special needs of women and children (Walsh 1977: 76–105). In the 1920s, the women physicians, social workers and public health nurses who ran the Sheppard-Towner clinics for maternal and child health in the United States were similarly carrying out what they saw as the special mandate of women health care professionals (Costin 1983). The current women's movement in the United States and Canada has also fostered women's health clinics and women-dominated medical institutions, but their goal is to restructure the delivery of services so that the physician is one of an egalitarian health care team, and the client is taught principles of self-help.[1]

Some women physicians may find the current women's health movement uncongenial to practicing the kind of medicine they have been trained for (Howell 1977). It is also logical that humane, client-oriented services be extended to men as well, and this goal might be better served by making common cause with like-minded male physicians than by working through separate women's groups. Women who want to be able to do productive work in the existing system will have to be influential enough to make reforms to support their priorities, and this aim takes group action. Men may be helpful, but it falls to women themselves to fight women's battles.

Working within the system:
emphasizing gender to undercut gender

The paradox of feminist politics is that women working in male-dominated institutions must form groups to attain the social power to challenge their treatment *as* a group. On her own, a woman is vulnerable to all the effects of informal discrimination – tracking into sex-appropriate work, devaluation of accomplishments, invisibility as a candidate for positions of authority, denigration for both commitment to and neglect of family responsibilities. Pursuing her career in isolation, a woman is likely to ignore the chilling effect of the gradual accumulation of the minutiae of informal discrimination. If she fights it on an informal level, she is labeled "abrasive." If she takes formal action against discriminatory practices, she is labeled "trouble-maker." As a group, women physicians can be very effective in many ways. During medical training, organizations of women faculty, students, and house staff can lobby to change sexist textbooks and lecture material and to revise curricula to better integrate women's perspectives. They can get child care, family living quarters and cafeteria arrangements and suggest ways of altering work schedules so that *all* house staff can have time to meet non-medical commitments. Women faculty can become mentors and role models for women physicians in training. And what is most important, senior women physicians can sponsor the career advancement of promising younger women.

Groups of women in office-based practices can form referral networks, coverage arrangements, and shared practices. In professional organizations, women's caucuses can insist on adequate representation of women on programs, committees, and in officerships. They can make sure that meetings are held at times that are manageable for those who have families but do not have a traditional wife at home. They can give each other the moral support to legitimize the time they spend on their "third job" – professional networking.

Women's committees in academic medical associations can serve as contacts for positions, suggest names for reviewing papers and grant proposals, for editorial boards and conference programs, and make sure that research women doctors are doing, that may not be in the mainstream, gets a fair share of funding and visibility. Within their own medical institutions, they can serve on promotion and search committees to make sure women candidates are looked for and considered seriously. They can bring class action discrimination suits for inequities in salaries. In cases of individual discrimination, they can bring pressure to bear on administrations in person and in letters, raise money, exchange information, go to the media, and offer necessary emotional support.

Women must be prepared to fight the system of gender discrimination for a long time. Gender inequities are pervasive and long-standing because they are built into social institutions and maintained by everyday assumptions about appropriate work for women and men in and out of the home. Gender discrimination cannot be countered by citing individual examples of women in their careers, or shared responsibilities at home. Personal solutions are vital for individuals to survive, but it takes concerted, politically sophisticated group action to restructure deeply embedded social arrangements. When women and men do the same kind of work in the same way and have the same responsibilities for home and family, gender as a social status will no longer be meaningful. If you think that would not be revolutionary, imagine a world without the social categories "man" and "woman".

The danger is that when women have succeeded in forming effective "old-girl" networks and in placing representative numbers of women in existing institutions, they will relax their efforts or disband entirely. Women will still need support from other women if they are not to be co-opted. In my view, the ultimate goal is not for women to join men in inner circles imbued with the male perspective on work, family life, and social service, but for the establishment of new values which reflect the needs and priorities of all members of society – female and male, old and young, rich and poor.

Note

1   See B.K. Rothman 1982; Young 1981; Marieskind 1980, 1975; Kleiber and Light 1978; Razek 1978; Marieskind and Ehrenreich 1975; Seaman 1975.

Appendix I
The AAMC Survey

My national sample of female and male physicians comes from the Association of Medical Colleges Longitudinal Survey of the Class of 1960 (Erdmann, R.F. Jones, and Tonesk, 1979). The respondents in this study attended seventy-seven United States medical schools, a sample selected by geographical region (northeast, southeast, north central, south central, west), by financial support (public and private), by stratifying the scores of entering freshmen on the Medical College Admission Test (MCAT), and by willingness to participate. Subjects were surveyed from the point of entry into medical school, in 1956, until 1976, or sixteen years after their expected graduation. The original sample consisted of 2,821 respondents, of whom 156 were women. The final number of respondents, as of 1976, was 1,850–1,750 men and 100 women.

For my sample, I matched the 100 female physicians who responded to the 1976 Longitudinal Survey Questionnaire with 300 male physicians, a number sufficient for stable estimates of gender differences. The following characteristics were used for matching: type of medical school attended (public or private), geographical region of medical school (northeast, southeast, north central, south central and west), and Medical College Admissions Test scores (verbal ability, quantitative ability, general information, science achievement). The MCAT scores were collapsed into one variable and categorized into high and low score groups on the basis of the median scores of female respondents. Matching on both school and MCAT scores at the same time controls for the effect of school attended as it interacts with the achievement potential of the student (Marshall, Fulton, Wesson 1978). My final sample from the AAMC Survey research study consists of 97 women and 291 men, since there were no males with matching characteristics for three of the women.

Age and race

There is no data on the age or race of the respondents, but the elimination of the black medical schools in the original sample implies that most of the subjects were white. If the respondents were in their early twenties when they entered medical school in 1956 (there were few late starters at that time), then it can be assumed that most were in their early forties in 1976.

Marital status and number of children

Among the 291 men, 88 per cent were married, 8 per cent were divorced or separated, 1 per cent were widowed and 3 per cent had never been married. Among the 97 women, 63 per cent were married, 14 per cent were divorced or separated, 4 per cent were widowed, and 19 per cent were never married. Of the men, 6 per cent had no children, another 6 per cent had one child, 27 per cent had two children, and 60 per cent had three or more children. There was no information from three of the men on this question. Of the women, 28 per cent had no children, 8 per cent had one child, 27 per cent had two children, and 37 per cent had three or more children.

Type of practice

Of the men, 60 per cent were in fee-for-service, 20 per cent in salaried, 4 per cent in group, and 3 per cent in contract practice. Four per cent were in miscellaneous other types of practice, and there was no answer from 8 per cent. Of the women, 34 per cent were in fee-for-service, 42 per cent in salaried, 3 per cent in group, and 1 per cent in contract practice. Two per cent were in other types of practice, and there was no answer from 12 per cent.

117

Specialties

The specialties ranged widely, with expected proportions of men and women in surgery (15 per cent to 2 per cent) and pediatrics (7 per cent to 23 per cent). Pediatrics was the most popular specialty for the women. The most popular specialty for the men was internal medicine; 19 per cent of the men and 13 per cent of the women listed it as their area of specialization. Ten per cent of the men and 6 per cent of the women said they were in general or family practice.

Appendix II
The interview study

I conducted face-to-face interviews in 1979 with physicians affiliated with the Department of Internal Medicine of a prestigious metropolitan medical center. All the women physicians in the department who were listed as active faculty members in 1978–79 and who were not solely involved in teaching and administration were solicited for interviews. Matches were found among male physicians by asking each woman physician to suggest a male physician she had trained or worked with. If the woman was married to a doctor in the Department of Medicine, as were seven, he was included in the sample as her match. The final number of usable interviews provided data on thirty-three women and thirty-one men.

Age, race, and national origin

Of the women, twenty-seven were graduates of US medical schools and six were graduates of foreign medical schools; of the men, twenty-six were US medical school graduates and five were foreign medical school graduates. One of the women and two of the men were black. All of the graduates of foreign medical schools were white, and two were from the United States. The respondents ranged in age from thirty to seventy-nine, and were fairly evenly divided by gender in each age cohort.

Marital status and number of children

At the time of the interview, twenty-one (64 per cent) of the women and twenty-seven (87 per cent) of the men were married; two of the men and one of the women were widowed, and one of the women was divorced. Of the women, seventeen were or had been married to physicians; of the men, ten had wives who were physicians. Of the married or formerly married men, three (10 per cent) had no children, four (14 per cent) had one child, fifteen (52 per cent) had two children, and seven (24 per cent) had three or more. Of the married or formerly married women, six (26 per cent) had no children, three (13 per cent) had one, seven (30 per cent) had two, and seven (30 per cent) had three or more.

Type of practice

Twenty-two of the sixty-four respondents were in primarily entrepreneurial careers (fee-for-service office practice). Of the forty hospital-based physicians, a little over half had academic careers (clinical research, teaching, and care of clinic patients), and the rest combined private practices with their hospital duties. The gender breakdown was fairly even for these three types of careers. Two additional women had institutional careers in nursing homes, schools, and employee health services, although some of the office-based physicians had at one time or another worked at these types of jobs.

Subspecialties

While all of the physicians interviewed were affiliated with the Department of Internal Medicine, they were in a variety of specialties, including dermatology, hematology, oncology, cardiology, and rehabilitation. They were located in three different hospitals and two research institutions that were part of the medical center. Those who were hospital-based were located in fifteen different units.

Appendix II

Physician couples

The interview sample included seventeen women and ten men who were or had been married to physicians, comprising twenty couples. I was able to interview both the husband and wife in seven couples. The husbands and wives in all but four of the twenty couples were about the same age, which meant they had gone through their career phases at the same time. In two cases, the husbands were about ten years older than their wives; in two cases, the husbands were a few years younger. The foreign medical school graduates were married to physicians who had gone to the same type of school.

In thirteen of the twenty couples, the husband and wife had the same type of career; eight of the couples were both in hospital-based careers for most of their working lives, and in five, both were in office practice. In four of the couples, the husband and wife had briefly shared a practice or an office at some point in their careers. In two of the couples, the husband and wife were in the same specialty, and in one they were also affiliated with the same medical center, but they worked in different buildings and used different names. Of the eight couples with the same institutional affiliation, half used different names. Eight of the couples had the same institutional affiliation, but were in different specialties. In half the couples, the husbands and wives were in different specialties and had different affiliations.

References

Ackerman-Ross, S. and Sochat, N. (1980) Close Encounters of the Medical Kind: Attitudes Toward Male and Female Physicians. *Social Science and Medicine* 14A: 60–4.

Adams, J. W. (1977) Patient Discrimination Against Women Physicians. *Journal of the American Medical Women's Association* 32: 255–61.

Ahern, N. C. and Scott, E. L. (1981) Career Outcomes in a Matched Sample of Men and Women Ph.D.s: An Analytical Report. Washington, D.C.: National Academy Press.

Angell, M. (1981) Women in Medicine: Beyond Prejudice. *New England Journal of Medicine* 304: 1161–163.

—— (1982) Juggling the Personal and Professional Life. *Journal of the American Medical Women's Association* 37: 64–8.

Aronson, S. G. (1974) Marriage with a Successful Woman: A Personal Viewpoint. In R. B. Kundsin (ed) *Women and Success: The Anatomy of Achievement*. New York: Morrow.

Bauder-Nishita, J. (1980) Gender-Specific Differentials of Medical Practice in California. *Women and Health* 5: 5–15.

Becker, H. S., Geer, B., Hughes, E. C., and Strauss, A. L. (1961) *Boys in White*. Chicago: University of Chicago Press.

Beil, C., Sisk, D. R., and Miller, W. E. (1980) A Comparison of Specialty Choices Among Senior Medical Students Using Bem

References

Sex-role Inventory Scale. *Journal of the American Medical Women's Association* 35: 178–81.

Berger, J., Cohen, B. P., and Zelditch Jr., M. (1972) Status Characteristics and Social Interaction. *American Sociological Review* 37: 241–55.

Berger, J., Fisek, M. H., Norman, R. Z., and Zelditch Jr., M. (1977) *Status Characteristics and Social Interaction: An Expectation States Approach*. New York: Elsevier.

Berman, E., Sacks, S., and Lief, H. (1977) The Two-Professional Marriage: A New Conflict Syndrome. In H. H. Frank (ed) *Women in the Organization*. Philadelphia: University of Pennsylvania Press.

Bernard, J. (1964) *Academic Women*. University Park: Pennsylvania State University Press.

—— (1981) *The Female World*. New York: Free Press.

Beuf, A. H. (1978) Women in Medicine: Better Studies Needed. *Annals of International Medicine* 88: 122–23.

Bewley, B. and Bewley, T. H. (1975) Hospital Doctors' Career Structure and Misuse of Medical Womanpower. *Lancet* 2 (9 August): 270–72.

Blackwell, E. (1977) *Pioneer Work in Opening the Medical Profession to Women*. New York: Schoken Books. (Originally published in 1895 by Longmans, Green, New York and London.)

Blackwell, J. E. (1981) *Mainstreaming Outsiders: The Production of Black Professionals*. Bayside, NY: General Hall.

Bloom, S. W. (1973) *Power and Dissent in Medical School*. New York: Free Press.

Bluestone, N. R. (1978) The Future Impact of Women Physicians on American Medicine. *American Journal of Public Health* 68: 760–63.

Blumberg, R. L. and Dwaraki, L. (1980) *India's Educated Women: Options and Constraints*. Delhi: Hindustan Publishing Corporation.

Bobula, J. D. (1980) Work Patterns, Practice Characteristics, and Incomes of Male and Female Physicians. *Journal of Medical Education* 55: 826–33.

Bourne, P. G. (1977) You Can't Use It, But Don't Lose It: Sex in Medical School. Proceedings, Conference on Women's Leadership and Authority in the Health Professions. Santa Cruz, Calif. 19–21 June.

—— (1979) Coping with Subtle Discrimination: The Catch-22 of Taking Action. Unpublished paper.

Bourne, P. G. and Wikler, N. J. (1978) Commitment and the Cultural Mandate: Women in Medicine. *Social Problems* 25: 430–40.

Braslow, J. B. and Heins, M. (1981) Women in Medical Education: A Decade of Change. *New England Journal of Medicine* 304: 1129–135.

Brown, S. and Klein, R. H. (1982) Woman-Power in the Medical Hierarchy. *Journal of the American Medical Women's Association* 37: 155–64.

Bryson, J. B. and Bryson, R. (1978) Dual-Career Couples. *Psychology of Women Quarterly* 3: 5–120.

Bucher, R. and Stelling, J. G. (1977) *Becoming Professional*. Beverly Hills, Calif.: Sage Publications.

Bullough, B. and Bullough, V. (1972) A Brief History of Medical Practice. In E. Freidson and J. Lorber (eds) *Medical Men and Their Work*. Chicago: Aldine-Atherton.

Bullough, V. and Voght, M. (1973) Women, Menstruation and Nineteenth Century Medicine. *Bulletin of the History of Medicine* 47: 66–82.

Carter, M. J. and Carter, S. B. (1981) Women's Recent Progress in the Professions or, Women Get a Ticket to Ride After the Gravy Train Has Left the Station. *Feminist Studies* 7: 477–504.

Cartwright, A. and Anderson, R. (1981) *General Practice Revisited*. New York: Methuen.

Cartwright, L. K. (1977) Continuity and Noncontinuity in the Careers of a Sample of Young Women Physicians. *Journal of the American Medical Women's Association* 32: 316–21.

Chaney, E. M. (1973) Old and New Feminists in Latin America: The Case of Peru and Chile. *Journal of Marriage and the Family* 35: 331–43.

Cohen, E. D. and Korper, S. P. (1976) Women in Medicine: A Survey of Professional Activities, Career Interruptions, and Conflict Resolutions. *Connecticut Medicine* 40: 103–10, 195–200.

Cole, J. R. (1979) *Fair Science: Women in the Scientific Community*. New York: Free Press.

Cole, S., Cole, J. R., and Simon, G. A. (1981) Chance and Consensus in Peer Review. *Science* 214: 881–86.

Coombs, R. H. (1978) *Mastering Medicine: Professional Socialization in Medical School*. New York: The Free Press.

Coser, R. L. (1981) Where Have All the Women Gone? In C. F. Epstein and R. L. Coser (eds) *Access to Power: Cross-National Studies of Women and Elites*. London: George Allen & Unwin.

Coser, R. L. and Rokoff, G. (1971) Women in the Occupational World: Social Disruption and Conflict. *Social Problems* 18: 535–54.

Costin, L. B. (1983) Women and Physicians: The 1930 White House Conference on Children. *Social Work*, March–April: 108–14.

Crane, D. (1972) *Invisible Colleges: Diffusion of Knowledge in Scientific Communities*. Chicago: University of Chicago Press.

References

Cuca, J. M. (1979) The Specialization and Career Preferences of Women and Men Recently Graduated from U.S. Medical Schools. *Journal of the American Medical Women's Association* 34: 425–35.

Daniels, M. J. (1960) Affect and Its Control in the Medical Intern. *American Journal of Sociology* 66: 259–67.

Davidson, L. R. (1975) *Sex Roles, Affect, and the Woman Physician: A Study of the Impact of Latent Social Identity Upon the Role of the Professional*. Ph.D. Dissertation. New York University.

—— (1978) Medical Immunity? Male Ideology and the Profession of Medicine. *Women and Health* 3: 3–10.

—— (1979) Choice by Constraint: The Selection and Function of Specialties Among Women Physicians-In-Training. *Journal of Health Politics, Policy and Law* 4: 200–20.

Dickerson, G. R. and Pearson, A. A. (1979) Sex Differences of Physicians in Relating to Dying Patients. *Journal of the American Medical Women's Association* 34: 45–7.

Dodge, N. (1971) Women in the Soviet Economy. In A. Theodore (ed) *The Professional Woman*. Cambridge, Mass.: Schenkman.

Drachman, V. (1976) *Women Doctors and the Women's Medical Movement: Feminism and Medicine 1850–1895*. Ph.D. Dissertation. State University of New York at Buffalo.

Ducker, D. G. (1978) Believed Suitability of Medical Specialties for Women Physicians. *Journal of the American Medical Women's Association* 33: 25–32.

—— (1980) The Effect of Two Sources of Role Strain on Women Physicians. *Sex Roles* 6: 549–59.

Edwards, A. L. (1953) *Manual for the EPPS* (Revised). New York: Psychology Corporation.

Ehrenreich, B. and English, D. (1973) *Witches, Midwives, and Nurses: A History of Women Healers*. Old Westbury, NY: Feminist Press.

Eisenberg, L. (1981) The Distaff of Aesculapius – The Married Woman as Physician. *Journal of the American Medical Women's Association* 36: 85–8.

Elston, M. A. (1977) Women in the Medical Profession: Whose Problem? In M. Stacey, M. Reid, C. Heath and R. Dingwall (eds) *Health and the Division of Labour*. London: Croom Helm.

—— (1980) Medicine: Half Our Future Doctors? In R. Silverstone and A. Ward (eds) *The Careers of Professional Women*. London: Croom Helm.

Engleman, E. G. (1974) Attitudes Toward Women Physicians: A

Study of 500 Clinic Patients. *Western Journal of Medicine* 120: 95–100.

Epstein, C. F. (1970a) Encountering the Male Establishment: Sex-Status Limits on Women's Careers in the Professions. *American Journal of Sociology* 75: 965–82.

—— (1970b) *Women's Place: Options and Limits in Professional Careers.* Berkeley: University of California Press.

—— (1974a) Ambiguity as Social Control: Consequences for the Integration of Women in Professional Elites. In P. L. Stewart and M. G. Canter (eds) *Varieties of Work Experience.* Cambridge, Mass.: Schenkman.

—— (1974b) Bringing Women In: Rewards, Punishments, and the Structure of Achievement. In R. B. Kundsin (ed) *Women and Success: The Anatomy of Achievement.* New York: Morrow.

—— (1981) *Women in Law.* New York: Basic Books.

Erdmann, J. B., Jones, R. F., and Tonesk, X. (1979) *AAMC Longitudinal Study of Medical School Graduates of 1960.* (DHEW Publication No. 79-3235) Hyattsville, Md.: National Center for Health Services Research.

Eskilon, A. and Wiley, M. G. (1976) Sex Composition and Leadership in Small Groups. *Sociometry* 39: 183–94.

Farrell, K., Witte, M. H., Holguin, M., and Lopez, S. (1979) Women Physicians in Medical Academia: A National Statistical Survey. *Journal of the American Medical Association* 241: 2808–812.

Fava, S. F. and Genovese, R. G. (1983) Family, Work, and Individual Development in Dual-Career Marriages: Issues for Research. In H. Z. Lopata and J. H. Pleck (eds) *Research in the Interweave of Social Roles: Families and Jobs* 3: 163–85.

Fennell, M. L., Barchas, P. R., Cohen, E. G., McMahon, A. M., and Hildebrand, P. (1978) An Alternative Perspective on Sex Differences in Organizational Settings: The Process of Legitimation. *Sex Roles* 4: 589–604.

Fesith, K. A. (1977) Office for Women in Medicine: A Model for Social Change. *Journal of Medical Education* 52: 928–30.

Fett, I. (1976) The Future of Women in Australian Medicine. *Medical Journal of Australia Special Supplement*, vol. 3. Greenwich, Conn.: JAI Press.

Fidell, L. S. (1980) Sex Role Stereotypes and the American Physician. *Psychology of Women Quarterly* 4: 313–30.

Fishman, D. B. and Zimet, C. N. (1972) Specialty Choice and Beliefs About Specialties Among Freshmen Medical Students. *Journal of Medical Education* 47: 524–33.

References

Fletcher, S. W. (1982) Women Physicians: Old Times or New Era? *The Pharos* 45: 2–9.

Fox, J. G. and Richards Jr., J. M. (1977) Physician Dominance and Location of Foreign and U.S. Trained Physicians. *Journal of Health and Social Behavior* 18: 366–75.

Fox, R. C. (1957) Training for Uncertainty. In R. K. Merton, G. Reader and P. Kendall (eds) *The Student Physician.* Cambridge, Mass.: Harvard University Press.

Frank, H. H. and Katcher, A. H. (1977) The Qualities of Leadership: How Male Medical Students Evaluate Their Female Peers. *Human Relations* 30: 403–16.

Freidson, E. (1960) Client Control and Medical Practice. *American Journal of Sociology* 65: 374–82.

—— (1970a) *Professional Dominance.* New York: Atherton.

—— (1970b) *Profession of Medicine.* New York: Dodd, Mead.

—— (1975) *Doctoring Together.* New York: Elsevier.

—— (1983) The Reorganization of the Profession by Regulation. *Law and Human Behavior* 7(2/3): 279–90.

Frey, H. (1980) Swedish Men and Women Doctors Compared. *Medical Education* 14: 143–53.

Fruen, M. A., Rothman, A. I., and Steiner, J. W. (1974) Comparison of Characteristics of Male and Female Medical School Applicants. *Journal of Medical Education* 49: 137–45.

Gallagher, E. B. and Searle, C. M. (1983) Women's Health Care: A Study of Islamic Society. In J. H. Morgan (ed) *Third World Medicine and Social Change.* Lanham, Md: University Press of America.

Garland, H. and Smith, G. B. (1981) Occupation Achievement Motivation as a Function of Biological Sex, Sex-Linked Personality, and Occupational Stereotypes. *Psychology of Women Quarterly* 5: 568–85.

Geyman, J. P. (1980) Increasing Number of Women in Family Practice: An Overdue Trend. *Journal of Family Practice* 10: 207–8.

Ginzberg, E. (1978) Women in Medicine: What is Really Happening. *Journal of Medical Education* 53: 843–44.

Goffman, E. (1983) The Interaction Order. *American Sociological Review* 48: 1–17.

Goldblatt, A. and Goldblatt, P. B. (1976) The Status of Women Physicians: A Comparison of USMG Women, USMG Men, and FMGs. *Journal of the American Medical Women's Association* 31: 325–28.

Goode, W. J. (1957) Community Within a Community: The Professions. *American Sociological Review* 22: 194–200.

127

—— (1982) Why Men Resist. In B. Thorne with M. Yalom (eds) *Rethinking the Family*. New York: Longman.

Granovetter, M. K. (1973) The Strength of Weak Ties. *American Journal of Sociology* 78: 1360–380.

—— (1974) *Getting a Job: A Study of Contacts and Careers*. Cambridge, Mass.: Harvard University Press.

Gray, R. M., Newman, W. R., and Reinhardt, A. M. (1966) The Effect of Medical Specialization on Physicians' Attitudes. *Journal of Health and Human Behavior* 7: 128–32.

Grenell, B. (1979) *Correlates of Specialty Choice of Female Medical Students*. Ph.D. Dissertation. Columbia University.

Grimm, J. W. and Stern, R. N. (1974) Sex Roles and Internal Labor Market Structures: The 'Female' Semi-Professions. *Social Problems* 21: 690–705.

Gross, W. and Cravitz, E. (1975) A Comparison of Medical Students' Attitudes Toward Women and Women Medical Students. *Journal of Medical Education* 50: 390–94.

Hall, F. S. and Hall, D. T. (1979) *The Two-Career Couple*. Reading, Mass.: Addison-Wesley.

Hall, O. (1946) The Informal Organization of the Medical Profession. *Canadian Journal of Economics and Political Science* 12: 30–41. Also in W. R. Scott and E. Volkart (eds) (1966) *Medical Care*. New York: Wiley.

—— (1948) The Stages of a Medical Career. *American Journal of Sociology* 53: 327–36.

—— (1949) Types of Medical Careers. *American Journal of Sociology* 55: 243–53.

Handy, C. (1978) Going Against the Grain: Working Couples and Greedy Occupations. In R. Rapoport and R. N. Rapoport (eds) *Working Couples*. New York: Harper & Row.

Harlin, V. (1981) The American Medical Women's Association and Today's Practicing Physician. *Connecticut Medicine* 45: 493–94.

Harris, B. J. (1978) *Beyond Her Sphere: Women and the Professions in American History*. Westport, Conn.: Greenwood Press.

Harris, M. B. and Conley-Muth, M. A. (1981) Sex Role Stereotypes and Medical Specialty Choice. *Journal of the American Medical Women's Association* 36: 245–52.

Haug, M. R. (1976) The Erosion of Professional Authority: A Cross-Cultural Inquiry in the Case of Physicians. *Health and Society* Winter: 83–106.

Hayes, M. D. (1981) The Impact of Women Physicians on Social

Change in Medicine: The Evolution of Humane Health Care Delivery Systems. *Journal of American Medical Women's Association* 36: 82–4.

Heins, M. (1979) Career and Life Patterns of Women and Men Physicians. In E. Shapiro and L. Lowenstein (eds) *Becoming a Physician: Development of Values and Attitudes in Medicine*. Cambridge, Mass.: Ballinger.

Heins, M. and Braslow, J. (1981) Women Doctors: Productivity in Great Britain and the United States. *Journal of Medical Education* 15: 53–6.

Heins, M., Hendricks, J., and Martindale, L. (1979) Attitudes of Women and Men Physicians. *American Journal of Public Health* 69: 1132–139.

Heins, M., Smock, S., Jacobs, J., and Stein, M. (1976) Productivity of Women Physicians. *Journal of the American Medical Association* 236: 1961–964.

Heins, M., Smock, S., Martindale, L., Jacobs, J. and Stein, M. (1977) Comparison of the Productivity of Women and Men Physicians. *Journal of the American Medical Association* 237: 2514–517.

Hilberman, E., Konac, J., Perez-Reyes, M., Hunter, R., Scagnelli, J., and Sanders, S. (1975) Support Groups for Women In Medical School: A First-Year Program. *Journal of Medical Education* 50: 867–75.

Holder, A. R. (1979) Women Physicians and Malpractice Suits. *Journal of the American Medical Women's Association* 34: 239–40.

Holmes, F. F., Holmes, G. E., and Hassanein, R. (1978) Performance of Male and Female Medical Students in a Medical Clerkship. *Journal of the American Medical Association* 239: 2259–262.

Holmstrom, L. L. (1972) *The Two-Career Family*. Cambridge, Mass.: Schenkman.

Horner, M. S. (1972) Toward an Understanding of Achievement-Related Conflicts in Women. *Journal of Social Issues* 28: 157–76.

Howell, M. C. (1974) Sounding Board: What Medical Schools Teach About Women. *New England Journal of Medicine* 291: 304–7.

—— (1975) A Woman's Health School? *Social Policy* 6 (Sept./Oct.): 50–3.

—— (1977) Guest Editorial: Can We Be Feminist Physicians? Mirages, Dilemmas and Traps. *Journal of Health Politics, Policy and Law* 2: 168–72.

Hubbard, R. (1977) On Constructing a Non-sexist Medical School Curriculum. The American Medical Women's Association Workshop for Women in Medical Academia. Tuscon, Ariz. 15–21 May.

Hughes, E. C. (1971) *The Sociological Eye*. Chicago: Aldine-Atherton.

Hughes, M. J. (1943) *Women Healers in Medieval Life and Literature*. New York: King's Crown Press.

Hummell, K. J., Kaupen-Hall, H., and Kaupen, W. (1970) The Referring of Patients as a Component of the Medical Interaction System. *Social Science and Medicine* 3: 597–607.

Humphreys, P. and Berger, J. (1981) Theoretical Consequences of the Status Characteristics Formulation. *American Journal of Sociology* 86: 953–83.

Hunt, J. G. and Hunt, L. L. (1977) Dilemmas and Contradictions of Status: The Case of the Dual-Career Family. *Social Problems* 24: 407–16.

Hunt, J. G. and Hunt, L. L. (1982) The Dualities of Careers and Families: New Integrations or New Polarizations? *Social Problems* 29: 499–510.

Hurd-Mead, K. C. (1931) Seven Important Periods in the Evolution of Women in Medicine. *Bulletin of the Medical Women's National Association* 35: 6–15.

Intons-Peterson, M. J. and Johnson, H. (1980) Sex Domination of Occupations and the Tendencies to Approach and Avoid Success and Failure. *Psychology of Women Quarterly* 4: 526–47.

Izraeli, D. N. (1983) Sex Effects or Structural Effects? An Empirical Test of Kanter's Theory of Proportions. *Social Forces* 62: 153–65.

Jeffreys, M., Gauvin, S., and Guleson, O. (1965) Comparison of Men and Women in Medical Training. *The Lancet* (June 26): 1381–383.

Johnson, D. G. and Sedlacek, W. E. (1975) Retention by Sex and Race of 1968–1972 U.S. Medical School Entrants. *Journal of Medical Education* 50: 925–33.

Jolly, P. (1981) Datagram: Women Physicians on U.S. Medical School Faculties. *Journal of Medical Education* 36: 151–53.

Jones, A. B. and Shapiro, E. C. (1979) The Peak of the Pyramid: Women in Dentistry, Medicine, and Veterinary Medicine. *Annals of the New York Academy of Sciences* 323: 79–91.

Jones, J. G. (1971) *Career Patterns of Women Physicians*. Ph.D. Dissertation. Brandeis University.

Jussim, J. and Muller, C. (1975) Medical Education for Women: How Good an Investment? *Journal of Medical Education* 50: 571–80.

References

Kanter, R. M. (1976) The Impact of Hierarchical Structures on the Work Behavior of Women and Men. *Social Problems* 23: 415–30.
—— (1977a) *Men and Women of the Corporation*. New York: Basic Books.
—— (1977b) Some Effects of Proportions on Group Life: Skewed Sex Ratios and Responses to Token Women. *American Journal of Sociology* 82: 965–90.
Kaufman, D. R. (1978) Associational Ties in Academe: Some Male and Female Differences. *Sex Roles* 4: 9–21.
Kaufman, D. R. and Richardson, B. L. (1982) *Achievement and Women: Challenging the Assumptions*. New York: Free Press.
Kehrer, B. H. (1976) Factors Affecting the Incomes of Men and Women Physicians. *Journal of Human Resources* 11: 526–45.
Kessler-Harris, A. (1982) *Out to Work: A History of Wage-Earning Women in the United States*. New York: Oxford.
Kleiber, N. and Light, L. (1978) *Caring for Ourselves: An Alternative Structure for Health Care*. Vancouver, Can.: University of British Columbia School of Nursing.
Kobrin, F. E. (1966) The American Midwife Controversy: A Crisis of Professionalization. *Bulletin of the History of Medicine* 40: 350–63.
Kosa, J. (1970) Entrepreneurship and Charisma in the Medical Profession. *Social Science and Medicine* 4: 25–40.
Kosa, J. and Coker, R. E., Jr. (1971) The Female Physician in Public Health: Conflict and Reconciliation of the Sex and Professional Roles. In A. Theodore (ed) *The Professional Woman*. Cambridge, Mass.: Schenkman.
Kutner, N. G. and Brogan, D. R. (1980) A Comparison of the Practice Orientations of Women and Men Students at Two Medical Schools. *Journal of the American Medical Women's Association* 35: 80–6.
Kutner, N. G. and Brogan, D. R. (1981) Problems of Colleagueship for Women Entering the Medical Profession. *Sex Roles* 7: 739–46.
Langwell, K. M. (1982) Differences by Sex in Economic Returns with Physician Specialization. *Journal of Health Politics, Policy and Law* 6: 752:61.
Lapidus, G. W. (1978) *Women in Soviet Society*. Berkeley: University of California Press.
Larson, M. S. (1977) *The Rise of Professionalism*. Berkeley: University of California Press.
Latour, B. and Woolgar, S. (1979) *Laboratory Life: The Social Construction of Scientific Facts*. Beverly Hills, Calif.: Sage.

131

Laws, J. L. (1975) The Psychology of Tokenism: An Analysis. *Sex Roles* 1: 51–67.

Leeson, J. and Gray, J. (1978) *Women and Medicine*. London: Tavistock.

Leserman, J. (1981) *Men and Women in Medical School*. New York: Praeger.

Levine, A. and Crumrine, J. (1975) Women and the Fear of Success: A Problem in Replication. *American Journal of Sociology* 80: 964–74.

Levinson, D. J. (1978) *The Seasons of a Man's Life*. New York: Ballantine.

Levinson, R. M., McCollum, K. T., and Kutner, N. G. (1984) Gender Homophily in Preferences for Physicians. *Sex Roles* 10: 315–25.

Levitt, J. (1977) Men and Women as Providers of Health Care. *Social Science and Medicine* 11: 395–98.

Lewin, M. (1982) Playing the Game – For Keeps. *Journal of the American Medical Women's Association* 37: 202–03.

Lin, N., Ensel, W. M., and Vaughn, J. C. (1981) Social Resources and Strength of Ties: Structural Factors in Occupational Status Attainment. *American Sociological Review* 46: 393–405.

Lin, N., Vaughn, J. C., and Ensel, W. M. (1981) Social Resources and Occupational Status Attainment. *Social Forces* 59: 1163–181.

Lipman-Blumen, J. (1976) Toward a Homosocial Theory of Sex Roles: An Explanation of the Sex Segregation of Social Institutions. *Signs* 1(3) Part 2: 15–31.

Lockheed, M. E. and Hall, K. P. (1976) Conceptualizing Sex as a Status Characteristic: Applications to Leadership Training Strategies. *Journal of Social Issues* 32: 111–24.

Lopate, C. (1968) *Women in Medicine*. Baltimore: The Johns Hopkins Press.

Lorber, J. (1975a) Women and Medical Sociology: Invisible Professionals and Ubiquitous Patients. In M. Millman and R. M. Kanter (eds) *Another Voice: Feminist Perspectives on Social Life and Social Science*. New York: Doubleday Anchor.

—— (1975b) Good Patients and Problem Patients: Conformity and Deviance in a General Hospital. *Journal of Health and Social Behavior* 16: 213–25.

—— (1979) Trust, Loyalty, and the Place of Women in the Informal Organization of Work. In J. Freeman (ed) *Women: A Feminist Perspective*. Palo Alto, Calif.: Mayfield Publishing Company. (Also in third edition 1984.)

References

—— (1981a) The Limits of Sponsorship for Women Physicians. *Journal of the American Medical Women's Association* 36: 329–38.

—— (1981b) Minimalist and Maximalist Feminist Ideologies and Strategies for Change. *Quarterly Journal of Ideology* 5: 61–66.

—— (1982) How Physicians Spouses Influence Each Other's Careers. *Journal of the American Medical Women's Association* 37: 21–26.

Lorber, J. and Ecker, M. (1983) Career Development of Female and Male Physicians. *Journal of Medical Education* 58: 447–56.

Lorber, J. and Satow, R. (1977) Creating a Company of Unequals: Sources of Occupational Stratification in a Ghetto Community Mental Health Center. *Sociology of Work and Occupations* 4: 281–302.

Lovelace, J. C. (1985) Career Satisfaction and Role Harmony in Afro-American Women Physicians. *Journal of the American Medical Women's Association* 40. In press.

Luke, R. D. and Thomson, M. A. (1980) Group Practice Affiliation and Interphysician Consulting Patterns Within a Community General Hospital. *Journal of Health and Social Behavior* 21: 334–44.

Lurie, E. (1981) Nurse Practitioners: Issues in Professional Socialization. *Journal of Health and Social Behavior* 22: 31–48.

Makosky, V. P. (1976) Sex-Role Compatibility of Task and of Competition, and Fear of Success as Variables Affecting Women's Performance. *Sex Roles* 2: 237–48.

Mandelbaum, D. R. (1978) Review Essay: Women in Medicine. *Signs* 4: 136–51.

—— (1981) *Work, Marriage and Motherhood: The Career Persistence of Female Physicians*. New York: Praeger.

Marieskind, H. I. (1975) Restructuring Ob-Gyn. *Social Policy* 6 (Sept./Oct.): 48–9.

—— (1980) *Women in the Health System*. St. Louis. Mo.: C. V. Mosby.

Marieskind, H. I. and Ehrenreich, B. (1975) Towards Socialist Medicine: The Women's Health Movement. *Social Policy* 6 (Sept./Oct.): 34–42.

Marrett, C. B. (1979) On the Evolution of Women's Medical Societies. *Bulletin of the History of Medicine* 53: 434–48.

—— (1980) Influences on the Rise of New Organizations: The Formation of Women's Medical Societies. *Administrative Science Quarterly* 25: 185–99.

Marshall, R. J., Fulton, J. P., and Wessen, A. F. (1978) Physician Career Outcomes and the Process of Medical Education. *Journal of Health and Social Behavior* 19: 124–38.

Martin, P. Y. (1982) "Fair Science: Test or Assertion?" A Response to Cole's "Women in Science." *Sociological Review* 30: 478–508.

Martin, P. Y. and Osmond, M. W. (1982) Gender and Exploitation: Resources, Structure, and Rewards in Cross-Sex Exchange. *Sociological Focus* 15: 403–16.

Matteson, M. T. and Smith, S. V. (1977) Selection of Medical Specialties: Preferences vs. Choices. *Journal of Medical Education* 52: 548–54.

McGrath, E. and Zimet, C. N. (1977a) Similarities and Predictors of Specialty Interest Among Female Medical Students. *Journal of the American Medical Women's Association* 32: 361–73.

McGrath, E. and Zimet, C. N. (1977b) Female and Male Medical Students: Differences in Specialty Choice Selection and Personality. *Journal of Medical Education* 52: 293–300.

McPherson, M. P. (1981) "On the Same Terms Precisely": The Women's Medical Fund and the Johns Hopkins School of Medicine. *Journal of the American Medical Women's Association* 36: 37–40.

Mechanic, D. (1976) *The Growth of Bureaucratic Medicine*. New York: Wiley.

Meeker, B. F. and Weitzel-O'Neill, P. A. (1977) Sex Roles and Interpersonal Behavior in Task-Oriented Groups. *American Sociological Review* 42: 91–105.

Merton, R. K. (1968) The Matthew Effect in Science. *Science* 159: 56–63.

Merton, R. K., Reader, G., and Kendall, P. (1957) *The Student-Physician*. Cambridge, Mass.: Harvard University Press.

Miller, A. E. (1977) The Changing Structure of the Medical Profession in Urban and Suburban Settings. *Social Science and Medicine* 11: 233–43.

Miller, J., Lincoln, J. R., and Olson, J. (1981) Rationality and Equity in Professional Networks: Gender and Race as Factors in the Stratification of Interorganizational Systems. *American Journal of Sociology* 87: 308–35.

Miller, S. J. (1970) *Prescription for Leadership: Training for the Medical Elite*. Chicago: Aldine.

Miller, S. M. (1971) On Men: The Making of a Confused Middle-Class Husband. *Social Policy* 2: 33–9.

Mitroff, I. (1974) *The Subjective Side of Science: A Philosophical Inquiry into the Psychology of the Apollo Moon Scientists*. New York: Elsevier.

Morais, H. M. (1976) *The History of the Afro-American in Medicine*. Cornwell Heights, Pa.: Publishers Agency.

Morantz, R. M. (1974) The Lady and Her Physician. In M. S. Hartman and L. Banner (eds) *Clio's Consciousness Raised: New Perspectives in the History of Women*. New York: Harper & Row.

References

—— (1978) The 'Connecting Link': The Case for the Woman Doctor in Nineteenth Century America. In J. W. Leavitt and R. L. Numbers (eds) *Sickness and Health in America*. Madison: University of Wisconsin Press.

—— (1982a) Feminism, Professionalism, and Germs: The Thought of Mary Putnam Jacobi and Elizabeth Blackwell. *American Quarterly* 34(5): 459–78.

—— (1982b) Introduction: From Art to Science: Women Physicians in American Medicine, 1600–1980. In R. M. Morantz, C. S. Pomerleau, and C. H. Fenichel (eds) *In Her Own Words: Oral Histories of Women Physicians*. Westport, Conn.: Greenwood Press.

Morantz, R. M. and Zschoche, S. (1980) Professionalism, Feminism, and Gender Roles: A Comparative Study of Nineteenth Century Medical Therapeutics. *Journal of American History* 68: 568–88.

Mumford, E. (1970) *Interns: From Students to Physicians*. Cambridge, Mass.: Harvard University Press.

Nadelson, C. C. and Nadelson, T. (1980) Dual-Career Marriages: Benefits and Costs. In F. Pepitone-Rockwell (ed) *Dual Careers*. Beverly Hills, Calif.: Sage.

Nadelson, C. C. and Notman, M. T. (1974) Success or Failure: Women as Medical School Applicants. *Journal of the American Medical Women's Association* 29: 167–72.

Nadelson, C. C., Notman, M. T., and Lowenstein, P. (1979) The Practice Patterns, Life Styles and Stresses of Women and Men Entering Medicine: A Follow-up Study of Harvard Medical School Graduates from 1967 to 1977. *Journal of the American Medical Women's Association* 34: 400–06.

Nadelson, T. and Eisenberg, L. (1977) The Successful Professional Woman: On Being Married to One. *American Journal of Psychiatry* 134: 1071–076.

Offe, C. (1977) Translated by J. Wickham. *Industry and Inequality*. New York: St Martins Press.

Olson, J. and Miller, J. (1983) Gender and Interaction in the Workplace. In H. Lopata and J. H. Pleck (eds) *Research in the Interweave of Social Roles: Jobs and Families*, vol. 3. Greenwich, Conn.: JAI Press.

Oppenheimer, C. K. (1977) The Sociology of Women's Economic Role in the Family. *American Sociological Review* 42: 387–406.

Ortiz, F. I. (1975) Women and Medicine: The Process of Professional Incorporation. *Journal of the American Medical Women's Association* 30: 18–30.

Osaka, M. M. (1978) Dilemmas of Japanese Professional Women. *Social Problems* 26: 15–25.

Papenek, H. (1971) Purdah in Pakistan: Seclusion and Modern Occupations for Women. *Journal of Marriage and The Family* 33: 517–30.

—— (1973) Men, Women, and Work: Reflections on the Two-Person Career. *American Journal of Sociology* 78: 852–72.

Pawluch, D. (1983) Transitions in Pediatrics: A Segmental Analysis. *Social Problems* 30: 449–65.

Pepitone-Rockwell, F. (ed) (1980) *Dual Careers*. Beverly Hills, Calif.: Sage.

Piliavin, J. A. (1976) On Feminine Self-Presentation in Groups. In J. J. Roberts (ed) *Beyond Intellectual Sexism: A New Woman, A New Reality*. New York: David McKay.

Piradova, M. D. (1976) USSR – Women Health Workers. *Women and Health* 1: 24–9.

Pleck, J. H. (1977) The Work-Family Role System. *Social Problems* 24: 417–27.

—— (1983) Husband's Paid Work and Family Roles. In H. Z. Lopata and J. H. Pleck (eds) *Research in the Interview of Social Roles: Families and Jobs*, vol. 3. Greenwich, Conn.: JAI Press.

Poll, C. (1978) *No Room at the Top: A Study of the Social Processes that Contribute to the Underrepresentation of Women on the Administrative Levels of the New York City School System*. Ph.D. Dissertation. The City University of New York.

Poloma, M. M. and Garland, T. N. (1971) The Myth of the Egalitarian Family: Familial Roles and the Professionally Employed Wife. In A. Theodore (ed) *The Professional Woman*. Cambridge, Mass.: Schenkman.

Pugh, M. D. and Wahrman, R. (1983) Neutralizing Sexism in Mixed-Sex Groups: Do Women Have to be Better than Men? *American Journal of Sociology* 88: 746–62.

Quadagno, J. S. (1976) Occupational Sex-Typing and Internal Labor Market Distributions: An Assessment of Medical Specialties. *Social Problems* 442–53.

—— (1978) Career Continuity and Retirement Plans of Men and Women Physicians: The Meaning of Disorderly Careers. *Sociology of Work and Occupations* 5: 55–74.

Rapoport, R. and Rapoport, R. (1976) *Dual-Career Families Re-examined*. New York: Harper & Row.

Rapoport, R. and Rapoport, R. (eds) (1978) *Working Couples*. New York: Harper & Row.

Relman, A. S. (1980) Here Come the Women. (Editorial) *New England Journal of Medicine* 302: 1252–253.

References

Reskin, B. F. (1978a) Sex Differentiation and the Social Organization of Science. *Sociological Inquiry* 48: 3–37.

—— (1978b) Scientific Productivity, Sex, and Location in the Institution of Science. *American Journal of Sociology* 83: 1235–243.

Rice, D. (1979) *Dual-Career Marriage: Conflict and Treatment.* New York: Free Press.

Rinke, C. M. (1981) The Professional Identities of Women Physicians. *Journal of the American Medical Association* 245: 2419–421.

Roeske, N. A. and Lake, K. (1977) Role Models for Women Medical Students. *Journal of Medical Education* 52: 459–66.

Romm, S. (1982) Woman Doctor in Search of a Job. *Journal of the American Medical Women's Association* 37: 11–15.

Roos, N. P., Gaumont, M., and Colwill, N. L. (1977) Female and Physician: A Sex Role Incongruity. *Journal of Medical Education* 52: 345–46.

Roos, P. A. (1983) Marriage and Women's Occupational Attainment in Cross-Cultural Perspective. *American Sociological Review* 48: 852–64.

Rosenthal, M. M. (1979) Perspectives on Women Physicians in the U.S.A. Through Cross-Cultural Comparison: England, Sweden, USSR. *International Journal of Women's Studies* 2: 528–40.

Rosenthal, P. A. and Eaton, J. (1982) Women MDs in America: 100 Years of Progress and Backlash. *Journal of the American Medical Women's Association* 37: 129–33.

Rosow, I. and Rose, K. D. (1972) Divorce Among Doctors. *Journal of Marriage and the Family* 34: 587–98.

Rossiter, M. W. (1982) *Women Scientists in America: Struggles and Strategies to 1940.* Baltimore: Johns Hopkins University Press.

Rothman, B. K. (1982) *In Labor: Women and Power in the Birthplace.* New York: W. W. Norton.

Rothman, S. M. (1978) *Woman's Proper Place.* New York: Basic Books.

Rothstein, W. G. (1972) *American Physicians in the 19th Century.* Baltimore: Johns Hopkins University Press.

Rowe, M. P. (1977a) Go Hire Yourself a Mentor. Proceedings, Conference on Women's Leadership and Authority in the Health Professions. Santa Cruz, Calif., 19–21 June.

—— (1977b) The Saturn's Rings Phenomenon: Micro-inequities and Unequal Opportunity in the American Economy. Proceedings, Conference on Women's Leadership and Authority in the Health Professions. Santa Cruz, Calif., 19–21 June.

Ruzek, S. B. (1978) *The Women's Health Movement*. New York: Praeger.

Scadron, A. (1980) AMWA's Experiment in Planned Change: A Report on the 'Women in Medical Academia' Project. *Journal of the American Medical Women's Association* 35: 299–301.

Scully, D. (1980) *Men Who Control Women's Health: The Miseducation of Obstetrician-Gynecologists*. Boston: Houghton Mifflin.

Seaman, B. (1975) Pelvic Autonomy: Four Proposals. *Social Policy* 6 (Sept./Oct.): 43–7.

Segovia, J. and Elinson, J. (1978) Sex Differences in Medical Practice in Argentina. *Social Science and Medicine* 12: 305–9.

Sennett, R. and Cobb, J. (1973) *The Hidden Injuries of Class*. New York: Vintage Press.

Shaffer, P. (1980) *Amadeus*. New York: Harper & Row.

Shapiro, E. C. and Jones, A. B. (1979) Women Physicians and the Exercise of Power and Authority in Health Care. In E. Shapiro and L. M. Lowenstein (eds) *Becoming a Physician: Development of Values and Attitudes in Medicine*. Cambridge, Mass.: Ballinger.

Shapley, D. (1974) Medical Education: Those Sexist Putdowns May Be Illegal. *Science* 184: 449–51.

Shortell, S. M. (1973) Patterns of Referral Among Internists in Private Practice: A Social Exchange Model. *Journal of Health and Social Behavior* 14: 335–48.

Shryock, R. H. (1966) Women in American Medicine. In *Medicine in America: Historical Essays*. Baltimore: Johns Hopkins University Press.

Shuval, J. T. (1983) *Newcomers and Colleagues. Soviet Immigrant Physicians in Israel*. Houston, Tex.: Cap and Gown Press.

Sidel, R. (1972) *Women and Child Care in China*. New York: Hill & Wang.

Skipper, J. K. and Gliebe, W. A. (1977) Forgotten Persons: Physicians' Wives and Their Influence on Medical Career Decisions. *Journal of Medical Education* 52: 764–66.

Smith-Rosenberg, C. and Rosenberg, C. (1973) The Female Animal: Medical and Biological Views of Women and Her Role in Nineteenth Century America. *Journal of American History* 60: 332–56.

Solomon, D. N. (1961) Ethnic and Class Differences Among Hospitals as Contingencies in Medical Careers. *American Journal of Sociology* 61: 463–71.

South, S. J., Bonjean, C. M., Corder, J., and Markham, W. T. (1982a) Sex and Power in the Federal Bureaucracy: A Comparative

References

Analysis of Male and Female Supervisors. *Work and Occupations* 9: 233–54.

South, S. J., Bonjean, C. M., Markham, W. T. and Corder, J. (1982b) Social Structure and Intergroup Interaction: Men and Women of the Federal Bureaucracy. *American Sociological Review* 47: 587–99.

Spangler, E., Gordon, M. A., and Pipkin, R. M. (1978) Token Women: An Empirical Test of Kanter's Hypothesis. *American Journal of Sociology* 84: 160–70.

Starr, P. (1982) *The Social Transformation of American Medicine.* New York: Basic Books.

Staver, S. (1983) Husband-Wife MDs. *American Medical News* 3 (18 Mar.): 36–7.

Stevens, R. A., Goodman, L. W., and Mick, S. S. (1974) What Happens to Foreign-Trained Doctors Who Come to the United States? *Inquiry* 11: 112–24.

Swafford, M. (1978) Sex Differences in Soviet Earnings. *American Sociological Review* 43: 657–73.

Symposium on the Academic Physician: An Endangered Species. (1981) *Bulletin of the New York Academy of Medicine* 57: 411–504.

Szasz, T. S. (1970) *The Manufacture of Madness.* New York: Dell.

Treiman, D. J. and Roos, P. A. (1983) Sex and Earnings in Industrial Society: A Nine-Nation Comparison. *American Journal of Sociology* 89: 616–50.

Tresemer, D. (1976) The Cumulative Record of Research on 'Fear of Success.' *Sex Roles* 2: 217–36.

—— (1977) *Fear of Success.* New York: Plenum.

Tuchman, G. (1980) Discriminating Science. *Social Policy* 11 (May/June): 59–64.

Wallace, H. M. (1980) Women in Medicine. *Journal of the American Medical Women's Association* 35: 201–11.

Wallis, L. A., Gilder, H., and Thaler, H. (1981) Advancement of Men and Women in Medical Academia: A Pilot Study. *Journal of the American Medical Association* 246: 2350–353.

Walsh, M. R. (1977) *"Doctors Wanted: No Women Need Apply" Sexual Barriers in the Medical Profession, 1835–1975.* New Haven, Conn.: Yale.

Ward, A. W. M. (1982) Careers of Medical Women. *British Medical Journal* 284: 31–3.

Webster, M. Jr. and Driskell, J. E. Jr. (1978) Status Generalizations: A Review and Some New Data. *American Sociological Review* 43: 220–36.

Weinberg, E. and Rooney, J. F. (1973) The Academic Performance of Women Students in Medical School. *Journal of Medical Education* 48: 240–47.

Weisman, C. S., Levine, D. M., Steinwachs, D. M., and Chase, G. A. (1980) Male and Female Physician Career Patterns: Specialty Choices and Graduate Training. *Journal of Medical Education* 55: 813–25.

Wertz, R. W. and Wertz, D. C. (1977) *Lying In: A History of Childbirth in America.* New York: Free Press.

Wikstrand-Westling, H., Monk, M. A., and Thomas, C. B. (1970) Some Characteristics Related to the Career Status of Women Physicians. *Johns Hopkins Medical Journal* 127: 273–86.

Williams, J. J. (1946) Patients and Prejudice: Lay Attitudes Toward Women Physicians. *American Journal of Sociology* 51: 283–87.

—— (1950) The Woman Physician's Dilemma. *Journal of Social Issues* 6: 38–44.

Williams, P. A. (1971) Women in Medicine: Some Themes and Variations. *Journal of Medical Education* 46: 584–91.

Williams, P. B. (1978) Recent Trends in the Productivity of Women and Men Physicians. *Journal of Medical Education* 53: 420–22.

Wilson, M. P. (1981) The Status of Women in Medicine: Background Data. *Journal of the American Medical Women's Association* 36: 62–79.

Wilson, M. P. and Jones, A. B. (1977) Career Patterns of Women in Medicine. Proceedings, Conference on Women's Leadership and Authority in the Health Professions, Santa Cruz, Calif., 19–21 June.

Witte, M. H. (1981) Death in an Untenured Position. (Editorial) *Journal of the American Medical Association* 246: 2356–357.

Witte, M. H., Arem, A. J., and Holguin, M. (1976) Women Physicians in United States Medical Schools: A Preliminary Report. *Journal of the American Medical Women's Association* 31: 211–13.

Wolf, W. C. and Fligstein, N. D. (1979a) Sex and Authority in the Workplace: The Causes of Sexual Inequality. *American Sociological Review* 44: 235–52.

Wolf, W. C. and Fligstein, N. D. (1979b) Sexual Stratification: Differences in Power in the Work Setting. *Social Forces* 58: 94–107.

Wolman, C. and Frank, H. (1975) The Solo Woman in a Professional Peer Group. *American Journal of Orthopsychiatry* 45: 164–71.

Wunderman, L. E. (1980) Female Physicians in the 1970s: Their Changing Roles in Medicine. In *Profile of Medical Practice.* Chicago: AMA Center for Health Services Research.

References

Yogev, S. (1982) Happiness in Dual-Career Couples: Changing Research, Changing Values. *Sex Roles* 8: 593–605.

Yohalem, A. M. (1979) *The Careers of Professional Women: Commitment and Conflict*. Montclair NJ: Allanheld/Universe.

Yokopenic, P. A., Bourque, L. B., and Brogan, D. (1975) Professional Communication Networks: A Case Study of Women in the American Public Health Association. *Social Problems* 22: 493–509.

Young, G. (1981) A Woman in Medicine: Reflections from the Inside. In H. Roberts (ed) *Women, Health and Reproduction*. London: Routledge & Kegan Paul.

Zimet, C. N. and Held, M. L. (1975) The Development of Views of Specialties During Four Years of Medical School. *Journal of Medical Education* 50: 157–66.

Zuckerman, H. (1977) *Scientific Elite: Nobel Laureates in the United States*. New York: Free Press.

Zuckerman, H. S. (1978) Structural Factors as Determinants of Career Patterns in Medicine. *Journal of Medical Education* 53: 453–63.

Name index

142

Name index

Name index

Mick, S. S. 51, 139
Miller, A. E. 14, 24, 51, 134
Miller, J. 9, 28, 134–35
Miller, S. J. 6, 32, 47, 66, 134
Miller, S. M. 91, 96, 134
Miller, W. E. 33, 123
Mitroff, I. 6, 134
Morais, H. M. 17, 134
Morantz, R. M. 2, 17–20, 112, 134–35
Muller, C. 14, 131
Mumford, E. 47, 135

Nadelson, C. C. 2, 14, 87, 135
Nadelson, T. 87, 98, 135
Newman, W. R. 32, 128
Norman, R. Z. 123
Notman, M. T. 2, 14, 135

Offe, C. 5, 135
Olson, J. 9, 28, 134–35
Oppenheimer, C. K. 84, 135
Ortiz, F. I. 78, 135
Osaka, M. M. 11, 135
Osmond, M. W. 11, 134

Papenek, H. 2, 95, 136
Pawluch, D. 28, 136
Pearson, A. A. 56, 125
Perez-Reyes, M. 129
Pepitone-Rockwell, F. 98, 136
Piliavin, J. A. 8, 136
Pipkin, R. M. 112, 139
Piradova, M. D. 2, 136
Pleck, J. H. 95–6, 136
Poll, C. 12, 112, 136
Poloma, M. M. 91, 96, 136
Pugh, M. D. 8, 14, 40, 136

Quadnagno, J. S. 1, 14, 33, 136

Rapoport, R. 98, 136
Reader, G. 47, 134
Reinhardt, A. M. 32, 128
Relman, A. S. 27, 78, 136
Reskin, B. F. 4, 11–12, 65, 68, 137
Rice, D. 98, 137
Richards, J. M. Jr 51, 106, 127
Richardson, B. L. 14, 131

Rinke, C. M. 47, 137
Roeske, N. A. 47, 137
Rokoff, G. 3, 11, 124
Romm, S. 71, 137
Rooney, J. F. 2, 140
Roos, N. P. 2, 137
Roos, P. A. 3, 16, 137
Rose, K. D. 80, 137
Rosenberg, C. 20, 138
Rosenthal, M. M. 2, 14, 136
Rosenthal, P. A. 29, 137
Rosow, I. 80, 137
Rossiter, M. W. 12, 15, 24, 137
Rothman, A. I. 2, 127
Rothman, B. K. 113, 137
Rothman, S. M. 23, 137
Rothstein, W. G. 18, 137
Rowe, M. P. 53, 109, 137
Ruzek, S. B. 2, 29, 113, 138

Sacks, S. 98, 123
Sanders, S. 129
Satow, R. 28, 133
Scadron, A. 63, 138
Scagnelli, J. 129
Scott, E. L. 14, 122
Scully, D. 41, 47, 138
Seaman, B. 113, 138
Searle, C. M. 2, 127
Sedlacek, W. E. 2, 130
Segovia, J. 2, 138
Sennett, R. 5, 138
Shaffer, P. 9–10, 138
Shakespeare, W. 29
Shapiro, E. C. 27, 29, 130, 138
Shapley, D. 39, 138
Shortell, S. M. 50, 138
Shryock, R. H. 2, 138
Shuval, J. T. 29, 138
Sidel, R. 97, 138
Simon, G. A. 6, 124
Sisk, D. R. 33, 123
Skipper, J. K. 88, 138
Smith, G. B. 14, 127
Smith, S. V. 33, 134
Smith-Rosenberg, C. 20, 138
Smock, S. 129
Sochat, N. 55, 122
Solomon, D. V. 6, 50, 138

145

Subject index

division of labor, by gender 95–7
double binds: of career women
11–12; of women physicians 41
Dual Doctor Families 98; *see also*
marriage

Edwards Personal Preference Schedule (EPPS) 44–5, 48, 125
England, and women physicians
25–6, 27
evaluation: differential 109; of peers
10, 44; and social characteristics
7–8
extraordinary accomplishments, as
method of advancement, 68–9

family responsibilities: 81–7; effects
of children 93–5
female professional networks 62–3
feminist movement 24; politics 111–
15; *see also* women's movement
future plans 104

gatekeepers, and colleague selection
6–8, 9–10, 31, 109
gender discrimination, and women
physicians 4, 6, 114; *see also* sex
discrimination
Gospel according to Matthew 5

homogeneity: of colleagues and patients 50; and gender 62; in
professional groups 5–6, 13; and
referrals 50
hospital: as focus of colleague community 58–9; setting up a practice
51–4

informal organization of medicine
50
inner circles 111; of practicing
physicians 14, 50, 62–3, 109, 115
interview study 119–21
Interns xi, 135

Johns Hopkins Medical School 20,
38

*Journal of the American Medical
Women's Association* 79
Julius Caesar 110

lay healers 17–18, 21
lucky breaks, as method of advancement 67–8

marital status: and AAMC survey
117; and physicians interviewed
83, 120; and professional productivity 2–3, 11, 43; and professional socializing 61, 92–3, 97; and
relative income of spouses 84–5
marriage: effects of 81–7; statistics
about 80–1; traditional 95; two
physician marriages 87–93
"marrying up" 80–1; or "Brahmin
effect" 81
Matthew effect 4–6, 12, 109
medical training: and achievement
42–7; pre-nineteenth century 17–
18; rewards during 2; and tracking 31–7
medicine: informal organization of
108–09; nineteenth century 18–
21, 112; pre-nineteenth century
17–18; twentieth century 21–5
mentors *see* role models; sponsorship
merit, and advancement 5–6
midwives 27–8

National Board of Medical Examiners (NBME) 43–6
National Health Service 24–5, 28
National Institutes of Health 102
New England Hospital for Women
and Children 19
nurse practitioners 27–8

office practice: acquiring patients
54–6; colleague community 57–
62; informal organization 50;
partnerships 53; referrals 49–50;
relationships with patients 56–7
older physicians, and work situation 100–02